ARBITRATION IN SUPPORTIVE PSYCHOTHERAPY AND COUNSELING

Professor Ashoka Jahnavi Prasad

1

Table of Contents

Figures and Tables

Many couples, families, doctors, lawyers, managers have used the process to reach decisions and solutions about the future direction of their relationships. These decisions reflect the participants' basic human needs for intimacy, connection, community, security, identity, equality, autonomy and recognition.

This is a highly rewarding process for the practitioner who provides a structure for clients and then "lets go" for them to "discover" the decisions that are right for them. At the end of five, six or eight sessions, participants usually reach the "ah-ha, now we know what has to happen, what needs to be done." Not just our clients, but their children, aging parents, or fellow employees benefit enormously when ambiguity and hostility are resolved.

I am deeply grateful to Cynthia Anderson LICSW, Rita Van Tassel LICSW, Jan

Schwartz Ed.D., Ruth Balser Ph.D., Judith Ashway LICSW, Lynne Yansen LICSW, Lu

Shurlan, LICSW for their technical inputs, support and encouragement during and

after the development of this process. To Paulette Speight, Ken LaKritz, M.D., Sally

Castleman, Janet Kurtz LICSW, Barbara Olson LICSW, Jeanne Kangas, Esq., Sarah and

Michael Dowling, Sarah

Smith and Souleymane Sagna, Meernoosh Watson, M.ED., Jane Bartrum LICSW, Les Wallerstein, Esq., Harry Manasiwich, Camilo Azcarate, JD, Frank Benson, MBA, Lisa Hoshmand Ph.D., Rick Reinkraut. Ph.D. and Carol Bonner, M.S.W, MBA., Justin Freed and The Program on Negotiation Forum, Mental Health Committee Members, and to each member of the Massachusetts Council on Family Mediation your support and encouragement have been invaluable.

I am very grateful to Judith Wallerstein who allowed me to liberally cite some of her research on the effects of separation and divorce on children and adolescents.

To Todd Wiseman, Annette Kurtz, my research associate and friend, and the late Alfred G. Meyer Ph.D., my mentor during my undergraduate years, I offer profound gratitude.

Last, but by no means least, to my mediation therapy

clients: You, with your wisdom, strength and creative resources have helped to build,

shape and change the mediation therapy process. In some of your deepest pain, you

have instructed me, and will be of service thereby to many other couples who later

walk in your shoes. To the many graduate students of mediation therapy-professional

social workers, counseling psychology students, psychologists, psychiatrists,

teachers, administrators, lawyers, nurses: You have dialogued, brainstormed, role-

played, challenged, and inspired me to broaden, deepen and fine tune the process of

mediation therapy so that it is much stronger and has wider applicability than when

originally conceived. This has been and will continue to be a challenging and

collaborative effort.

Why Mediation Therapy?

Mediation Therapy is designed specifically to address situations of conflict between close members of a family. Their goals for a therapeutic intervention may lie at nearly opposite ends of a continuum. One person wants to salvage the marriage, the other to divorce; one person wants to marry tomorrow, the other in five years and is still questioning with whom. A husband wants to build an addition to the home so his mother can live there, while his wife wants to find an excellent senior citizens' condominium for her. These conflicts in desires often elicit emotions that, if not reckoned with, may lead to inappropriate, even dangerous action.

At its optimum usefulness, mediation therapy is for people who cannot agree upon *anything.* Rarely, however, is this the case. The goal of mediation therapy is not consensus, or even partial agreement, between people. The goal is for each participant to gain genuine understanding of and acknowledge the other's way of seeing. This understanding of how the other person hears, perceives, and understands is what leads to a *mutual* decision about the future of the relationship or a successful resolution of the problem at hand. This enhanced, nonadversarial understanding is the sole goal of mediation therapy.

Couples and families who enter mediation therapy may or may not have a relationship disturbance or mental illness. If diagnostic assessment reveals disorders that can either be worked with or worked around in mediation therapy, then a mediation therapist can make a contract for mediation therapy with that couple. If, however, there are disorders such as those discussed in chapter 9, Selection of Clients, then alternative recommendations for treatment are advised.

Most couples who come for mediation therapy, regardless of mental illness or relationship disturbance, have in common feelings of confusion and ambivalence—of being in limbo and at wits' end. Nonetheless, is an entirely new therapeutic approach warranted for couples at their wits' end? And if so, why give this therapeutic intervention the name of *mediation*?

Is a New Therapy Necessary?

Why can't couples and families simply use one of the traditional processes already available to couples and families in trouble—for example, couples therapy, family therapy, or marriage counseling—in their decision making about the future?

Clients certainly can and do use these interventions to reach a decision regarding the future direction of their relationship or to successfully resolve a problem at hand. However there may be an inherent bias in the views of clinicians and clients alike, that the goals and purposes of marriage counseling and couples therapy are such things as

improving communication

overcoming specific problems such as parenting

disagreement, sexual difficulties, and money differences

helping the couple to differentiate from one another and

from their families of origin

These goals imply the working out of issues *within* the relationship, and, accordingly, imply a less than neutral bias or perspective about the future direction of the relationship.

When I have informally polled students in classes on mediation therapy, only a very few mention decision making about the relationship itself, or assessment of the relationship's future, as goals of couples therapy. More mention decision making in conjunction with marriage counseling than with couples therapy. The traditional therapeutic approaches for couples take a broad focus and may not always bring people to definitive decisions. By contrast, mediation therapy takes a narrow focus, with a single goal: to bring a couple to a decision.

A far less implicit, less subtle bias is the view expressed many years ago by Henry Grunebaum, Judith Christ, and Norman Nieburg in a paper about differential diagnosis: "If there is a serious question as to the marriage continuing or if one partner has more or less decided that the marriage will not continue, it is an almost certain indication that any form of couple treatment such as conjoint or concurrent therapy should not be considered."[1] Numerous clients enter my office each year after having been told by the psychotherapist they have consulted recently, by their health maintenance organization, or by their community health center, that their marital problems cannot be treated unless they are both committed to their marriage.

There are explicit proscriptions against using couples therapy to treat certain couples: those in which the partners' goals are different, or in which one or both partners are uncommitted or indecisive. Combined with the implicit bias toward saving the relationship that is often associated with marriage counseling or couples therapy, the creation of a specialized intervention for decision making becomes not only necessary, but urgent, if the needs of growing numbers of couples and families in crisis are to be adequately met.

At a time of marital upheaval, or of relationship or family crisis, people frequently are tempted to view and experience themselves as victims. Feeling "done to" and feeling taken advantage of, they drift into feeling more and more passive, vulnerable, out of control, or dependent; or they become ill. A strong positive feature of mediation therapy is that the attitudes and strategies of this intervention foster the progression of egofunctioning (what I term *mastery*), not regression. Mediation therapy strategies encourage people to take charge of themselves by giving them tasks to do, and by helping them to see themselves as experts on themselves, working in partnership with an expert on decision making. Psychotherapeutic interventions that purposefully promote a regressive transference (in which the psychotherapist is seen as an authority, rather than an expert) may inadvertently accentuate the feelings of helplessness, powerlessness, and victimization that people in this particular life-stage are experiencing.

Some psychotherapeutic circles assume that if a couple may be separating, they should see separate psychotherapists—in order to decide about the marriage in the privacy of their own thoughts and convictions about themselves and their mate. This assumption is diametrically opposed to the one that mediation therapy makes: couples deserve the option of having a calm, rational forum in which, together, they can come to terms with their futures. Increasingly, people are also using mediation therapy to make decisions about living together or getting married, as well as for other vitally important decisions about the future.

Whether a couple is deciding to marry, to divorce, to live together, to separate, to send a child to residential school or a parent to a senior citizens' home, there is most often present a palpable level of tension, conflict, anxiety, and ambivalence. It is these people with intense conflicts who are the chosen population for mediation therapy; and these are the same people who, according to the article on differential diagnosis cited above, are not appropriate for couples therapy. Writing twentytwo years ago, Grunebaum, Christ, and Nieburg stated, "Indeed, a therapist may be wise, depending on his inclinations, not to become involved in treatment with two spouses who in turn are intensely in conflict, or fully involved with one another."[2] Again, these are the same couples who can be well served by the process of mediation therapy.

As a highly cognitive but many-faceted approach to conflict negotiation, mediation therapy is tailor-made for couples and families in intense conflict. Although other psychotherapeutic approaches can and do help couples make decisions about their relationships, mediation therapy is the wrench designed to unscrew the locked nut of ambivalence about the future direction of relationships. The tools of couples therapy and marriage counseling may not always quite fit the need to make decisions about the future of a relationship. They may not have built-in specific techniques for conflict negotiation and decision making, and may not be able to accommodate families in intense conflict and those families whose members may have radically different goals for the intervention.

Why Give This Approach the Name of Mediation?

To mediate literally means to occupy a middle or mediating position. Psychotherapy often implies a process of selfunderstanding, which may or may not lead to character or behavior modification, to further personal growth, or to maturation. When psychotherapy is done with couples, there is the hope that it may contribute to improvement in the relationship. Mediation therapy, however, is not committed, as such, to any of these goals; they do seem to occur frequently and paradoxically, as by-products of the intervention. So *psychotherapy* is not a wholly accurate name for this focused decision-making process.

In mediation therapy, a neutral professional therapist sits in the middle position between two or more related persons in crisis, facilitating their decision making. Since many people who come to the process also have a diagnosable mental illness or relationship disturbance, the facilitator needs to be trained both as a mediator with ample skills to help people negotiate conflict, and as a psychotherapy clinician with advanced skills and experience. The combination of mediation and psychotherapy, together with conflict negotiation, defines to a large degree the process used in helping couples reach decisions. Hence, the name *mediation therapy: short-term decision making for couples and families in crisis.*

The name *mediation therapy* may be confused with divorce mediation, whose goal is a written agreement that becomes the basis for a couple's divorce settlement. The confusion of terms is both understandable and unfortunate. The general public is not yet clear about how or when divorce mediation is used, nor about how it differs from and compares with other methods for obtaining a divorce. Over time there has evolved a greater understanding of divorce mediation as a consensual approach for obtaining a divorce. I hope and anticipate that over time mediation therapy will be perceived as a distinct decisionmaking, therapeutic process, totally separate and very different from nontherapeutic divorce mediation.

Clients involved in the process of divorce mediation frequently ask whether the part of the process that focuses on discussion of the needs of their children is not actually a mental health intervention. The best interests of the children often are discussed in therapeutic interventions as well, but with different goals. In divorce mediation the ultimate goal of the discussion of the children's needs is to generate a consensus about the children's best interests, to be written into the agreement of the terms of a couple's divorce.

Divorce mediation is *not* psychotherapy and is *not* the decision-making process of mediation therapy. Each of these interventions has discrete and different goals. Though a couple may discover through mediation therapy a need or desire to separate or divorce, that discovery does not turn the process into divorce mediation—a new, separate process whose goal is the working out of the actual terms of the divorce settlement. If, during mediation therapy, a couple reaches a decision to divorce or separate, it is expected that a period of time will elapse before they are ready to choose negotiation, litigation, or mediation as the appropriate process for working out the terms of their separation or divorce agreement.

How is Mediation Therapy Similar to and Different from Other Approaches?

As already mentioned, mediation therapy is a therapeutic intervention and is not the same as the nontherapeutic process of divorce mediation. How, then, is it similar to and different from other therapeutic interventions?

Like James Mann's *Time-Limited Psychotherapy*, mediation therapy offers couples a time-limited process—typically twelve sessions. During the process, the members of the couple will make observations of themselves and of their relationships; express powerful emotions to one another; and learn skills in assertiveness, communication, negotiation, disagreement, and decision making, which ultimately will enable them to discover an important decision.

Since mediation therapy creates more intimacy between people during a time period when some individuals are desirous of far less contact (let alone intimacy), and since the process may or may not unleash the expression of painful emotions, the time limit offers an ending, with a decision made, as the motivation to endure more intimacy, more contact, and possibly more pain. The time limit brings a formal conclusion to being in limbo, an end to the indecision, as well as an ending of the relationship as it was. The time limit makes possible a mutual decision and a new form of relationship. It implies that having an indefinite amount of time available does not necessarily contribute to reaching a decision. The time limit also marks a formal beginning of a new way of life.

In common with psychoeducational approaches, mediation therapy involves instruction. It is an approach in which written material—papers, charts, books, as well as research findings— are shared with clients.

In some psychotherapies, clinicians are urged to be valuefree in their work with clients. In mediation therapy an open, direct partnership between expert and client is more useful than a reserved stance. The mediation therapist is, in fact, encouraged to share his or her values about child-rearing, marriage, divorce, and nonmarriage openly with clients. Among my values, which are shared from time to time with clients, are the following:

· The behavior and needs of any children of the couple

need to be considered during the decision-making process.

· Marriage is positively regarded by the mediation

therapist. I believe that marriage should not be casually dissolved in response to temporary reactions (a death in the family, for instance, or an anniversary, an illness, a birth, or the like.)

· Although divorce may be better for one or both adults,

there are indications that a relationship that causes parents great unhappiness and pain may nonetheless provide a context in which children are quite happy. Therefore, I believe that a wellconsidered divorce should be carried out with as much finesse, support, and caring for the children —and for one another—as possible.

· The mediation therapist is carefully trained to be *neutral*,

not siding with either individual, but with the best, most mutual decision the couple can make.

Other values held by the mediation therapist are shared with the couple

when the mediation therapist becomes aware of

26

the pertinence of the values to the discussion. Especially when the mediation therapist's values seem authoritative or definitive, they are shared *to minimize the risk of their blocking the mediation process.* The members of the couple are likewise encouraged to share their values and beliefs with each other and to respect the other's values even when they disagree with these values. (Ways of clarifying one's values and biases are discussed in chapter 2.)

Who Needs Mediation Therapy?

An important question arises at this point. How many couples, how many families will use and benefit from this decision-making approach? Some current speculation on expectations of marriage is that even couples who have good economic and parenting partnerships, but who feel they lack satisfying emotional relationships, now consider terminating their marriages. According to some reports fifty percent of recent marriages can be expected to end in divorce. Thirty-eight percent of children born in the mid-1980s will experience parental divorce before they are eighteen.[3] As the families who comprise these statistics grope for satisfactory solutions, the result will be marital crisis and indecision, with the disruptive ramifications extending to these individuals' ability to concentrate and be fully productive, at work and at home.

Far from contributing to a high divorce rate (which existed long before mediation therapy was invented), the mediation therapy approach provides a safe, calm, rational forum in which already indecisive couples can discover the best alternative for themselves and for their families.

As stated earlier, a growing number of not-yet-married couples come to mediation therapy to decide whether or not to be married, or whether or not to live together and when. Statistics are lacking for how many people could use mediation therapy to answer their questions about their relationship direction. Nevertheless, the fifty percent reported divorce rate for first marriages indicates that great numbers of people could use a rational, sane decision-making process to assess the advisability of marriage before the ceremony takes place, rather than afterward, at a time when dissatisfaction has set in.

In addition to its usefulness for couple relationships, many clinicians who have studied mediation therapy have indicated that their intended use of the process is to aid middle-aged people in making decisions about the future of their aging, sick, or terminally ill parents; or in making decisions about the residence and schooling of special needs children or young adults. Others have become mediation therapists in order to mediate conflicts between patients and their families during inpatient psychiatric hospitalization. Still other mediation therapists use the process to work out agreements between young people and their parents.

According to some reports, the two-parent family living together with their children is no longer likely to be the norm in the 1990s. The number of two-parent households declined from forty percent of all households in 1970 to twenty-seven percent in 1988 according to the U.S. Census Bureau's "Report on Families and Households."[4] It seems clear that people are making decisions toward family forms that they hope will suit them better than the long-established family forms to which they previously subscribed.

In 1987 a major U.S. newspaper editor declined to publish information about mediation therapy, reportedly because she felt this information would contribute to a higher divorce rate. On the contrary, it is clear that people have been making divorce decisions in great numbers without the benefit of mediation therapy. Mediation therapy, with its structured, rational, timelimited approach, is one of the best vehicles available for providing a safe and sane environment within which adults may make the wisest decisions of which they are capable. Some couples who would have divorced find a place to address their differences and stay married. Many who would have separated and divorced acrimoniously are able to "own" their decision together, feeling

mutually responsible for it; in mediation therapy one person does not assume all

the guilt with the other assuming a "done to" or "done in" posture. Some couples

decide not to marry after all, and some stage their living together and marriage

commitments over time. Some families build additions to their homes for an aging

parent, where that makes sense, while some acknowledge sooner rather than later

that a senior citizens' condominium, nursing home, or medical care facility is the

wiser placement. Decisions made in mediation therapy are based upon a couple's or

family's expression of and understanding of one another's issues, viewpoints, and

emotions.

Around the U.S. in the 1970s—from Los Angeles, to Atlanta, New York, Washington

D.C., Boston, and beyond—divorce mediation seemed to be welcomed in many

professional circles as an ancient idea whose time had come. Contrary to this arrival

of an old idea captured for divorce purposes, mediation therapy grew up pragmatically and developed inductively. A blend of techniques from

mediation, conflict negotiation, time-limited psychotherapy, and elsewhere was

implemented in its use with couples in crisis and has continuously evolved from

1979-1990.

Unlike divorce mediation (a new alternative to the old problem of getting a

divorce), mediation therapy does not arrive as a wholly new method. In *Problem-

Solving Therapy,* Jay Haley presents a pragmatic, problem-focused approach for

working with families. It is different from mediation therapy in not being specifically

focused for making a single discrete decision. Nonetheless, there is much in his

approach, as there is in Margot Fanger's possibility-focused approach, that echoes

the pragmatic, positive, forward-looking aspects of mediation therapy.

The theoretical framework for mediation therapy grew from the bottom up. An

integrated theoretical model has grown from the practical premises, attitudes, and

techniques, blended

together to become mediation therapy.

As a psychodynamically trained clinician simultaneously educated in family systems theory, and later trained in divorce and family mediation, I see mediation therapy as a blended approach.

Some clinicians learning mediation therapy have frequently described it as a cognitive approach. Other clinicians describe it as a structural or systems approach, or a psychoeducational approach. It has been called both a decision-making approach and a psychospiritual approach. Theoretically and strategically, the methods used are a blend of techniques from mediation, communications, family systems, and conflict negotiation theories, with ideas from decision-making theory and from neurolinguistic programming. This eclectic combination of many sources is intended to enrich rather than to dilute mediation therapy.

The techniques available for use in mediation therapy blend with the couple's current agenda at each session to become a living process of decision making. That the couple has come through the door requesting mediation therapy means that well over half the task is already accomplished in most cases: the couple has decided to make a decision.

The mediation therapist, from the outset, encourages the individuals to tolerate "not knowing" for a limited period of time, in the interest of making a wise decision. He or she often repeats throughout the intervention, that deciding may be a matter of uncovering a decision that is already deep within the individual but that he or she has not allowed him or herself to know up to this point.

The couple understands that explicit decision making as well as the urgency to know a decision will be suspended while the expression of strong emotions takes place. They understand, too, that stepping back for a systematic, rational overview of themselves as individuals and as a unit will also take place. A sharp increase in the couple's observations, information, and understanding of themselves takes place quickly in mediation therapy, together with the unleashing of long pent-up emotions. Becoming attuned to themselves, while observing themselves and their relationship, permits each individual to have a clearer vision of areas in which he or she needs to work, or it may make clear that further work in this relationship will most likely be unproductive.

Some individuals or couples will protest that marriages or relationships are based upon emotions and that rationality has no place in this arena. The mediation therapist agrees that emotions are just as vital as rationality, but that both need to be "equal guests" in the decision-making intervention.

The rational overview, or the head component in mediation

therapy, combines with the heart component, the sharing of deep emotion, to yield a deeper knowing within each individual of what is actually wanted in a relationship and what is available or potential in a particular relationship.

Often people expect to be able to make a decision based on the head component alone. In mediation therapy, an individual is frequently caught between two options, unable to make a decision based solely on rational thought. The person's eyes appear opaque and move from side to side, as if she or he is considering each option in turn: for example, "Shall I get a divorce? Or shall I stay married?" The person's eyes jump from right to left as if watching an imaginary tennis game in which the ball is being hit back and forth between the two choices.

In this match neither side will triumph. The volley will continue endlessly as long as the individual uses only reasoning, or the head component. Instead, a deeper knowing may be achieved by encouraging an individual to consider not only the head component but also emotional, educational, and sensory information. By changing the rules of the game, insisting that additional information be considered, I, as a mediation therapist, attempt to turn obsessive thinkers into farmers. That is my own metaphor for decision making as a "field of dreams." In the movie by that name, a farmer plows under his corn fields to build a baseball diamond and await some baseball players who were his father's heroes. The field may be seen as a metaphor for the farmer's eventual acceptance of his father. The field in mediation therapy then may be seen as a metaphor for the individual who accepts information to use in growing a decision.

In the field of mediation therapy the seeds of rational thought are planted. Seeds of sensory information and instructional information about communication, negotiation, disagreement, decision making, and assertiveness are also planted. The mediation therapist tends the fields with basic conflict negotiation attitudes and techniques. When the time is right and information has crosspollinated, an integrated understanding grows into an "Ah-ha! I understand now. I *know."* This blending of various types of information combined with deft conflict management by the mediation therapist virtually always leads to individuals growing decisions through integrated understanding. These individually grown decisions will then be negotiated with the partner's decision to become the collective decision of the couple or family. In mediation therapy, the process of deciding engages the head, the heart, the eyes, the ears, the intuition, and the inner source of wisdom within each individual—all of the senses and resources one has, not merely the rational resources.

The mediation therapist has faith in the process of helping people "know," and conveys her or his faith in the process to those who want to clarify their futures. Believing in the process, the mediation therapist describes it to them, what it is, how and why it works, and begins to guide them through what will be their own unique process. No two couples need explore their relationship or express their emotions in exactly the same way or at the same point in the mediation therapy process. In fact, it is better to talk about each couple's process, rather than about the mediation therapy process. Cues as to what new processes need to be created or employed with a couple are derived from the couple itself. Likewise, the cues that strong emotion needs to be expressed will frequently come from the individuals. And often indications about which exercises are needed, which questions may be asked and at what point, will come from the couple. For example, some couples will need to clue the therapist in on details of their families of origin before talking about their theories of the breakdown or impasse in their relationship. Other couples may need to reverse the order, or may need not to engage those questions at all. Nearly always, the mediation therapist allows the couple to lead if they have points of departure but is prepared to lead them and guide them if they do not have an agenda.

Some clinicians learning the mediation therapy process have asked for a description of the sessions from number one to number twelve   (see appendix A for such a description).

Mediation therapy could be and indeed has been well conducted in a sequential, predictable ordering of sessions. In this manner mediation therapy is predictable, duplicable, and efficient.

The artistic nature of the process of mediation therapy includes helping each couple to design their own process, based upon what is pressing for them to deal with; on their abilities to use visual, auditory, kinesthetic metaphor, and imagery; and on their defensive adaptations, their timing, and their character styles, among other factors. Allowing the initiative and control to come at times from the mediation therapist and at times from the couple requires that the mediation therapist be confident about the universality of the issues occurring in couples in crisis.

When the couple leads into or around a particular issue, the experienced mediation therapist will see how that issue dovetails with areas the therapist intends to include in the process. The artful application of the process involves letting go of control of the process at times, and picking up strong control at other times and, of course, the wisdom to know when to give structure to the process and when the couple needs to bring forward burning concerns, issues, and themes of their own.

Not all techniques, structures, attitudes that are introduced in this book, will be used with every couple. Other techniques will be used with every couple: in fact, a few techniques will be used at virtually the same time in every mediation therapy.

Attitudes that the mediation therapist brings to the process are likely to be the same with most couples and are crucial for setting a tone for decision making.

It is critical for the mediation therapist to believe that no matter how intense the conflict, how large the war, how ambivalent the parties, or how stagnant the relationship, those couples who have presented themselves to you to make a decision will be able to arrive at a mutual or mutually understood decision about their future direction. It is also important to realize that there are exceptions to this important rule.

Through her or his attitude, the mediation therapist needs to convey to the couple that she or he will be in charge of the process, including when to offer the couple control of the process. At the same time the couple is completely in charge of the decision they will be making. In conduct, the mediation therapist demonstrates to the couple that her or his function as an expert, in partnership with the two of them, is the antithesis of an authority who will decide their futures for them or pass judgment on them or on their relationship. As an expert, the mediation therapist guides the couple in catching a glimpse of themselves and in holding on to it long enough for each one to evaluate what he or she sees.

Through demeanor and actions the mediation therapist conveys that she or he is both empowering the couple to take charge of their lives and promoting their executive egofunctioning at its highest level, rather than tapping into regressive ego-functioning.

Typically, a mediation therapy session blends some of the following elements, which will be discussed fully in later chapters:

the couple's agenda,

some education about communication,

exercises to help them gain a rational overview of the relationship,

the sharing of strong emotions, negotiation of one or more conflicts,

education about assertiveness, conflict resolution, decision making, and effective disagreement.

Strategies, or *rational structures* as I call them, for helping the couple take a rational overview of their relationship are at the heart of the intervention. Delineated in chapter 4, the structures include pertinent questions to the couple, techniques and positions for the mediation therapist, and areas of knowledge to teach to couples.

At its most successful, mediation therapy helps people let go of denial and distortions about the self and about the relationship. It helps couples see clearly what they want and need personally and in a good long-term relationship; and it helps individuals see clearly what is actually available and what is potentially available in their relationship. In mediation therapy a decision about the future direction of the relationship is seen, discovered, or uncovered, based upon the confrontation of myriad actual facts and partisan perceptions about the relationship, and by sharing powerfully intense feelings. There is no need to "make" a decision through obsessional review: "Should I or shouldn't I get together, stay together, or have my parent or child live away in a residential placement?" The keys for "getting to know," for unlocking an internally congruent decision in mediation therapy, are: patience, tolerance of ambiguity, and the immense courage to peel away denial and distortions about the self and the relationship.

Notes

[1] Grunebaum, Christ, and Nieburg, "Differential Diagnosis," 6.

[2] Ibid., 8.

[3] Norton and Moorman, "Current Trends in Marriage and Divorce Among American Women," 3-14.

[4]

The Mediation Therapy Agreement:

Shaping the Process

The Initial Phone Calls

Prior to the initial session with a couple, you will have spoken first with one member of a couple on the telephone, then with the other member, who will have telephoned for a followup conversation with you. This symmetrical balance is necessary for the mediation therapist and necessary for the couple to begin the process with neutrality.

If the second member of the couple has been unable, for reasons of timing or location, to phone prior to the initial session, the mediation therapist should without question begin the initial session by stating that the first member of the couple has had the opportunity to speak with the mediation therapist to make the appointment and has had the opportunity to make inquiries about the process and the therapist; what questions, then, if any, does the second member of the couple have?

A demonstration of evenhandedness and symmetry is a cornerstone of the mediation therapy process. Talking with both members of a couple is not an occasional occurrence but one that needs to take place each and every time a new family is seen as well as throughout the intervention. Having spoken with only one member of a couple, the other may view you as hired by the partner and as somehow biased toward the person with whom the mediation therapist spoke.

In addition, I believe there is no human way of beginning and maintaining a neutral stance toward a couple except by speaking with both of them. Ideally, individuals will simply call to make an appointment, having already heard about mediation therapy and thus needing no further explanation of the process. Increasingly, couples call having heard of mediation therapy from friends or colleagues. For many others who call for couples work, the mediation therapist briefly describes some of the differences between couples therapy, marriage counseling, and mediation therapy, and asks the individual to describe the goal he or she wishes to accomplish during the course of the intervention. If you practice marriage counseling or couples therapy, it is not recommended that you attempt to convert every couple you treat into short-term decision-making candidates, but instead that you discriminate carefully those who are appropriate for a specific, structured decision-making approach. Fortunately, it doesn't usually seem to be a complicated process for the initial caller to identify what kind of intervention is appropriate for his or her needs.

In the process of the initial call, the caller has inevitably given you a thumbnail sketch of the situation, flavored with his or her perspective. If the caller has defined his or her needs as needing decision making, you will ask that the other partner be in telephone contact with you so that he or she may hear the *same* information, ask you questions and give you information. 48

You may suggest that if the two of them seem likely to want to make an appointment that they agree on some mutually available times. When the partner then calls, you will at that time be able to make an appointment. Frequently, the second partner will call you within fifteen minutes of the request to do so.

It is important that each partner choose the mediation therapist and mediation therapy process for him or herself, rather than merely accept the recommendations of a partner, a person with whom he or she may not be on the best of terms at this particular point in time. In *Problem-Solving Therapy* Jay Haley states, "Whenever one sees [I add, talks with] a person alone, the tendency is to join that person against others ... if the therapist joins one side against the other, he or she becomes part of the problem rather than part of the solution."[1] It behooves a therapist not to become a part of a couple's problem before they even enter the office.

—

Is this rule—that you speak to both members of a couple on

the telephone—a rule for its own sake? Talking with both members of the couple is a necessary precursor to the intervention that is to follow. This procedure does not vary; unless there are exceptional circumstances, it always takes place.

From the point of view of the calling parties, the function of their each speaking with the mediation therapist is manifold. The callers will have understood that the mediation therapist, from the very beginning of the process, is disciplined to be as neutral as possible between them, listening to both of them and instructing both of them equally about the process, so they may each choose the process independently of the other. If they have mentioned areas in which they are intensely angry with one another, some of that anger will have been defused by talking before the sessions have begun. Assuring that each individual has been heard effectively lessens the likelihood that one of them will enter the office for the first time with competitive hackles aroused to tell his or her side of the story. If the mediation therapist were to speak with only one member of the couple, the other would have the right to be suspicious about what had been said about him or her. The initial telephone call with you, the mediation therapist, during which you indicate that you are a sympathetic human being, albeit one who highly structures the conversation, may also decrease suspicion of you.

In the initial phone call, you may also ask the caller what, at this point, his or her personal goals are for any therapeutic intervention. This question relays to the caller that it is to be a unique intervention; only they as individuals know what it is that they need to accomplish. The question empowers the couple to begin actively engaging in their own process. The two-part telephone appointment setting, a single positioning action to establish neutrality and symmetry at the outset of the intervention, is equivalent in importance to many later positioning actions. The symmetrical telephone call is a graceful, effective means of leading into and shaping the process of mediation therapy; it overtly demonstrates the mediation therapist's commitment to neutrality and to recurring symmetrical input from each member of a couple or family. In abiding by a few invariable rules—such as talking with both members of a couple on the telephone before commencing mediation therapy—a basic tone, a general attitude, and a fundamental structure are set up for the entire process. People frequently comment about how differently things are done in mediation therapy from what they have heretofore experienced.

After the initial phone call, the attitudes and values that you, as the facilitator, bring are as important as any of the techniques for practicing mediation therapy. Both attitudes and techniques are needed in order to develop and preserve a neutral stance in the process of conducting mediation therapy and to strike an unwritten, good faith contract or mediation therapy agreement with your clients.

A major attitude or belief necessary for the development of neutrality is that it is necessary and appropriate for you to structure or even to control the process but not the outcome of mediation   therapy. The psychoanalytic approach to psychotherapy favors the psychotherapist's specifying the structure and thereby exercising control by indicating to the clients/patients that they should talk freely while the psychotherapist listens and comments or interprets occasionally. The mediation therapy approach indicates a different process: one in which the therapist is overtly in charge and in which she or he will balance the interaction between all participants. Many therapists have been trained in a listening process without needing to take charge or structure a smallgroup situation. To practice mediation therapy successfully, you will need to learn to do couples, family, or small-group work in order to become comfortable in taking an active, structuring role in the process. For structural, strategic, systemic family therapists, marriage counselors, couples therapists, and undoubtedly others, the transition to being clearly in charge in an active mode will not be as difficult as for those clinicians whose experience is in a psychoanalytic mode with individual patients. Becoming

comfortable in structuring the process is a necessity for you as mediation therapist.

The Couple's Goals

In most cases, as mediation therapist, you will want to begin the initial

session by repeating or initially calling for each individual's goals for the

intervention (As discussed later on, this is rational structure number one.). Sharing

their personal goals separates the individuals from the morass of interpersonal

issues between them. It individuates them out of the "coupleship. " In addition,

beginning with the individuals' goals precludes beginning the process with blaming.

In an initial session, I tell the couple that, in my eleven years' of experience with

mediation therapy, only one-third of couples have had the same goal to achieve—

that is, both

wanting to make a decision about the relationship. Two-thirds of all couples have had very different goals. In the following examples, both partners achieved their goals, which were different. One man's goal was to become less angry about his wife's leaving the country for several years without talking with him about the decision. His wife's goal was to decide upon returning to the United States whether there was any basis for trying to resume living together again. At the end of the mediation therapy he had become significantly less angry, and the couple had decided to divorce. Another man's goal was to try to see whether there was anything salvageable in his marriage, while his wife definitely wanted the man she had chosen for life to return home after he had been living away. That couple (the Andrews, cited in chapter 6), has since continued to be rewardingly married, but not without conflicts, for over ten years since the completion of mediation therapy.

It is important for couples to have their goals out on the table so the goals are crystal clear. You may share with them that it is more likely that each of them will achieve his or her own goal when the goals are known and not hidden from one another. How many instances can therapists think of where a single individual's goals are spoken of as the goal for both of the individuals? Eventually the first person feels betrayed because his or her partner's goal was never the same as the one that was taken or assumed as being a common goal. Better to allow it to be known from the outset that one person is undecided, ambivalent, or out-and-out negative about the relationship than to have this information uncovered at the end of the process. Through long experience, I have discovered the eminent workability of a couple's having two very different goals for a single process and their reaching mutually satisfactory conclusions to their differing goals. Indeed, if the couple has identical goals, they *may* not need to be engaged in the mediation process, which was specifically designed for couples in high conflict, and for those who are highly ambivalent or painfully undecided.

I emphasize that both individuals may achieve their goals, even if divergent, within the same intervention. The question often arises: is this the case even where one partner wants unequivocally to divorce and the other desperately wants to save the marriage? Sometimes. Through the process of mediation therapy, both people will uncover their personal needs and goals and hear those of their partner. They will take an in-depth look at the interaction of their various needs and fully explore their relationship with one another and with the wider world. So, while a decision to divorce may remain the dominant decision (that is, the ruling decision in the case where a decision is not mutual), both people will have, at a minimum, a far greater understanding of how the decision came to be made. In many cases, the decisions will be mutually *understood,* if not mutually made, and may even be accepted by both parties. Or, in certain cases it has, at times, been helpful to acknowledge that the decision is not mutual, but instead the decision of only one of the parties.

In directing the process in the initial session to the individual's goals, the mediation therapist is accomplishing many things. The importance of symmetry is reinforced by asking each individual what he or she needs to accomplish in a therapeutic intervention. Neither member of the couple should be allowed to dominate the intervention. An implicit message in this rational structure is that there are individual needs, perspectives, and goals—at this point the therapist is not asking them, as a unit, what they want to accomplish. He or she is individuating them: accepting each of them as an individual. The therapist begins the process, not by listening to them fight or watching them perform their ritual dance, but, instead, by demonstrating through questioning that they are not one ego mass but two individuals with unique goals. They must listen to one another, then be encouraged to hear the divergence as well as the similarities in their goals. By example, the therapist demonstrates that she or he will relieve them of the burden of structuring the process or of speaking for their mate: the therapist is clearly in charge of the process.

The Couple's Agenda

Most sessions, other than the first one, are best begun by asking the couple if either of them has issues on the front burner or items they would like to put on the agenda for that session. One opening is, "I have some items to discuss today, but I would like to start with where you are." One reason why people seem to respond favorably to this opening is that even if they were not aware of what they needed to take up in the session, the prospect of having their agenda pushed aside by a long-winded mediation therapist brings their concerns suddenly into focus. Or the mediation therapist can ask them whether they have been thinking about or having feelings about issues that arose in the last session? Have they talked about issues in a new way since they last saw you?

It is important to convey to the couple at all times that their concerns will be interwoven with the structured process of mediation therapy. There will be sessions during which all formal decision-making structures are suspended and many other sessions where the structures are nicely interwoven into the fabric of the couple's or family's current concerns.

Being at the fulcrum of the interaction is important for the mediation therapist. The fulcrum is the point where the chaotic energy of the couple is transferred into energy that constructively moves the couple ahead. Initially, conflict is high and anger deep.

Paraphrasing

Some mediation therapists may want to see for themselves, at the outset, the miscommunications, ritual dances, or maladaptiveness of communication, but rarely, do I find these helpful at the beginning of the process. Instead of allowing the couple to step immediately into their maladaptive communication with its attendant frustration and diminished self-esteem, I often

substitute the *paraphrase* at the beginning of the intervention. That is, most of the

initial dialogue in a session will be between me and the individuals. I then translate

and interpret, or paraphrase, information intended for each individual. Through

paraphrasing (rephrasing a statement for clarity), the poison or toxins can be taken

out of what one person is trying to convey to the other. The core of the message may

be conveyed from one partner to the other. Perhaps the most important tool of the

process, paraphrasing enables the therapist to cull the essence of what one member

is trying to convey and to present it in a rational, objective fashion, while checking

with the speaker as to whether he or she is being accurately represented. This then

helps the individuals remain individuated while they communicate with one

another. Paraphrasing is one of the most important techniques for maintaining a

neutral stance. In addition, many times a *metacommunication,* or implied

communication, is included with

the paraphrase. For example: "Your wife is desperate to have you share your feelings with her." Being desperate was in the wife's tone not her content, but it is nonetheless relayed as a part of the paraphrase.

Blaming and accusing the other person are literally outlawed in mediation therapy. From the outset of the intervention, the couple is encouraged to make "I" statements about how the other person's behavior makes an impact on him or her, rather than using blaming or accusing. This kind of instruction is sometimes necessary even during the initial statement of the couple's goals. Drawing-room politeness on the part of the mediation therapist is not in order—these initial moves to set clear, firm limits are necessary preparations for the conduct of the process.

To this point in the initial session the mediation therapist has demonstrated evenhandedness and neutrality. Each of the individuals has spoken about his or her personal goals. The therapist has made clear to the couple that they should speak for themselves without blame or accusation and has helped them learn to ensure that the partner has fully heard what they are saying.

The Contract Decision

At the end of an initial session, the therapist can often determine if the couple is appropriate to benefit from the mediation therapy process. People who have secrets bring challenges to the mediation therapy. Others who may well have serious difficulty using the mediation therapy process are families in which alcohol is a central issue. Those who manifest paranoia or any disordered thought processes or suspiciousness, those who have untreated affective or mood disorders, or the more primitive of the personality or character disorders need critical evaluation. People need healthy observing ego functions to be able to see themselves somewhat objectively. That isn't to say that some couples with a member with active alcoholism or a difficult personality disorder have not used the process productively. Yet, on balance, it requires so much more effort on the part of the clinician that a primary treatment for the condition or illness itself should be the first order of business. On the other hand, the predictability of the structure, combined with its controlled manageability, may provide the safety for some individuals or couples who might have difficulty in lessstructured settings. The beneficent overall structure of mediation therapy discussed in chapter 3 may provide a needed umbrella for weak ego structures not otherwise able to use a conjoint or a couple approach.

Once you have decided whether or not a couple is appropriate for the approach, and they have decided that the intervention is appropriate for them, you will want to think together with them about the frequency and duration of the meetings. Twelve weekly seventy-five minute sessions are an ideal number for the process, but due to time constraints or advanced personal stages in the decision-making process, it may be conducted in eight or ten sessions. Many people have used six, two-hour sessions

productively. One couple whose members lived in two different states conducted their

entire mediation therapy over the telephone, without meeting the mediation

therapist in person, in six, one-and-one- half-hour sessions. Other people know

they want to make a decision at the end of the year or summer and so choose a time

limit in that way. Most couples will know at least by the beginning of the second

session how many sessions seem appropriate for them. People seem to appreciate

being included in the decision-making loop involving the length of the contract. The

mediation therapy contract time limit may be renegotiated and extended toward the

end of the process; however, the benefits of such renegotiation don't always

supersede the drawbacks: more time may not be more beneficial than the

constructive, mobilizing anxiety built into the predetermined time limit.

Clients sometimes ask whether a different contract can be made at the end

of their twelve sessions: for example, a new

contract to help the family or a couple to grieve the breakup of the family and move onward after a decision to separate has been made; or a contract to help them implement their commitment to continue working on the relationship; or to implement a different decision, such as building an addition to the home for an aging parent.

The decision-making intervention is best done as a discrete process, with a beginning, a middle, and an end. From my experience I have come to believe that a break in time should be taken before any couples work, uncoupling work, or implementation work is undertaken. Generally speaking, these other post-mediation therapy interventions are less structured than mediation therapy. The structure of mediation therapy needs to be put behind both the clinician and the clients before another type of psychotherapy is begun. In addition, if you practice divorce mediation, ethical and practical considerations of performing a nontherapeutic intervention (divorce mediation) and a therapeutic intervention (mediation therapy) with the same couple prohibit you from engaging in nontherapeutic divorce mediation with mediation therapy clients.

Eleven years of specialized experience with couples who were able to make rational, mutual decisions about their own or a family member's future has led me to the conviction that couples and families, when adequately supported, can make some of the most difficult decisions of their lives *together*, without bitterness and grossly negative ramifications. It is appropriate for a mediation therapist to convey the results of his or her experiences with other couples and families to new families beginning the process. Conveying an attitude of hope for them, belief in them, and confidence in their abilities to reach a mutually understood decision helps them positively view the process of mediation therapy. In turn, this positive viewpoint generates positive physiological reactions for the therapist and the clients.

The Couple's Theories about Their Impasse

In the beginning of mediation therapy, I see couples needing more structure than later on in the process. It might seem logical to open up each individual's unique concerns after the goals for the process have been shared; however my experience is that an open- ended question at the beginning of the process is like letting the horses out of the gate before the race is scheduled to begin. Rather than asking an open-ended question, the mediation therapist may follow up the statement of the couple's goals by asking each of them what his or her *theory* is about the breakup or the impasse in the relationship, adding "you needn't be right"; (this is rational structure number two). As stated so well in *Women's Ways of Knowing,* "Theories become not truth, but models for approximating experience."[2] In other words, there is no one truth as to why the relationship broke down: only two people's experiences. Perhaps this question to elicit theories about the impasse or breakdown in the relationship helps individuals to recognize multi- causal contributors to their difficulties. The questioning may lead to a realization: "Maybe my perception is too simple or has more facets than I thought." Theories are unique and run the gamut:

"Our communication was never good, but broke down
completely when the baby was born ... or when he lost his job ... or when she had the affair."

"We struggle for control over everything and our power
struggles begin before we get out of bed in the morning. "

"We married for the wrong reasons, and the marriage was
broken before it began."

"She has all the money, which makes me feel inadequate."

There is an excellent opportunity after each member shares a theory to check out with the other person how he or she hears that theory and how it is viewed. This theory-talk keeps the focus on the cause of the difficulties rather than on blaming the other person. The question may imply hope if things were seen as better at an earlier time.

During this agreement formation stage, when the couple is deciding on a process, the first two rational structures (described in chapter 4) are presented to the client couple— individuals' goals for the intervention and their theories about the relationship's impasse or breakdown. The goals of these initial structures are:

1. to enlist the clients' full participation in the process 2. to engage

their creative thinking processes
3. to shape a process guided by their individual self
understanding and appreciation.

Couples don't make decisions; individuals do. Inquiring about the individuals' goals and theories begins to delineate the rational structures. (A more detailed discussion of the question, "What is your theory about the impasse or breakdown in your relationship?" occurs in chapter 4.) As with other rational structures, in the question about theory, the medium or the form of the question is often the biggest message: requesting individual theories implies that there is no one truth, but several evaluations of together- experiences.

The Therapist's Values

So far, I have discussed how it is that one might lead a couple into the process of mediation therapy, some techniques for gaining and/or preserving neutrality with the couples and families with whom you work, and the first two rational structures of the process: individuals' goals for the intervention and their theories about the relationship's impasse or breakdown. In addition, attitudes and values that a mediation therapist brings to the process are as important as actual concrete techniques to achieve balance, symmetry, and neutrality.

In developing a neutral stance the mediation therapist needs to have experience in understanding that two oppositional positions may both be true at the same time.

Getting to Yes by Roger Fisher and William Ury and *Getting Together* by Fisher and Scott Brown can help the beginning mediation therapist understand that reality lies not in one objective version of the truth but in how each person views a situation. These two books (and others listed in the bibliography) provide an important preliminary to the practice of mediation therapy. Another means to develop a neutral stance or attitude prior to practicing mediation therapy is by using a *bias sorter*, a series of questions such as the ones in the accompanying sidebars that help describe or delineate one's biases regarding relationships or other important topics. This is only one of a myriad of methods therapists need to apply in order to become aware of biases. Only by being aware of one's biases can one prevent their interference with the necessary neutral stance of mediation therapy. In *Problem- Solving Therapy,* Jay Haley states, "Simply not giving advice to a couple will not avoid the issue, since what the therapist thinks will be communicated somehow. It is preferable to clarify one's own thinking so that the marital problem does not meet an expert too confused and uncertain to be helpful." Haley further states, "As a therapist intervenes, he or she finds that a philosophy of life and marriage is necessary as a guide. The therapist must think through the issues of separation and divorce as well as responsibilities within the family group. The therapist's problem is how to keep [her or his] own biases from intruding into the changes sought by the couple."[3]

—

Each mediation therapist will want to develop her or his own bias sorters, depending either upon the idiosyncrasies of the client population seen, or upon her or his own idiosyncrasies. How can we realize or understand the attitudes and values we carry? A values and attitudes bias sorter such as the one listed in the accompanying box is one point of departure. Examining one's values, attitudes, and biases conjointly with a colleague or peer group is advised before attempting to practice mediation therapy. (Additional bias sorters are found in appendix C.)

1.   Do you believe in marriage? What is it?

            What is commitment? Are they the same?

2.   Do you believe in marital separation?

            Under certain circumstances? And not under other

            circumstances?

3.   Do you believe in divorce? Under

            certain circumstances and not under others?

4.   What religious, cultural, general

            background views, past and present, do you hold

            about divorce or marriage?

5.   When couples have children, does that

at all influence your opinion about whether
couples should stay together?

6.   Do children fare better in intact families
with unhappily married couples than in
divorced families with happily divorced
parents?

7.   How do you feel about gay and lesbian
relationships?   Are you at all
uncomfortable in the presence of these couples?

8.   How do you feel about interracial or
intercultural relationships (for example, a black
man and a white woman; a Russian man and an
American woman)? Are you uncomfortable in the
presence of these couples?

9.   How do you feel about relationships in

        which there is a large difference in age?

10.   How do you feel about relationships in

        which one person has a physical handicap, a

        mental disability, or AIDS?

11.   What is your own current image of a

        healthy relationship?

12.   Do you believe in living together on a

        long-term or short-term basis without

        marriage?

Bias Sorter: Conflict

1.   Do you like or enjoy conflict?

2.   Do you hate or avoid conflict?

3.   Is it easier to help others manage their

       conflicts than for you to deal directly with your own

       conflicts?

4.   How did your family of origin handle

       conflict?

5.   How much more effectively do you want

       to handle conflict between yourself and others,

       personally and professionally?

No one is without bias. In an intervention in which the neutrality of the clinician is

vital, it is important that the clinician be aware of his or her biases, values, and

attitudes. Acknowledging what these biases are goes a long way toward keeping them

in check and prevents them from unconsciously influencing a couple. At the extreme,

you might discover, as one student of mediation therapy did, that her strongly held

religious views prohibiting divorce made it impossible for her to take a neutral stand. She decided she could not apply the mediation therapy model with married couples needing to make a decision about the future direction of their relationship, although she could facilitate their discussions in other types of decisions. Another clinician discovered that he was exceedingly uncomfortable with anyone leaving a relationship with an AIDS patient. That he could not be neutral in helping partners, one of whom had AIDS, led that clinician not to attempt to use the approach with these clients. Another clinician discovered that growing up in the South where interracial marriages were prohibited kept her from being neutral about the future direction of the relationships of interracial couples. Still another clinician encountered a couple with an eighteen-year age difference. Her own marriage, with a large age difference, had broken up in the recent past with, from her point of view, age difference one of the significant contributing factors. In this case, however, the clinician's heightened awareness of her bias helped preserve her neutrality. The couple she was working with was able to share a monumental amount of rage with one another and made the decision

to marry. Although one can work with or around some biases, it is important to

disqualify oneself from attempting to work in decision-making areas where particular

bias buttons are pushed.

The Use of Individual Sessions

Generally speaking, mediation therapy clients are best served by being

seen together as a unit. That is because the purpose of the intervention is to provide a

sane setting within which people may together make one of the most important

decisions of their lifetimes. If individuals need a session (or sessions) alone to speak,

for example, about fears of a partner's homosexuality, or their own marital infidelity,

they typically ask during the initial phone call for an individual session. I usually tell

clients that individual sessions are not routine in the process, but are necessary in

some specific cases.

Unless a couple can *specifically* say that they don't need all information to be shared, I tell couples I will caringly and diplomatically share information when they cannot do so themselves from solo sessions in the next joint session. An example of an agreed upon translation from an individual session: "Carl, your wife is very concerned about your feelings. There is something that has been a secret, but that you may have sensed. It is a little more complicated than her simply being involved with someone else. That person is someone you know well, and you may well find a strange companion. That person is Linda's best friend, Margaret, with whom she is romantically involved." Out of sharing secret, delicate information, a process may unfold that includes trying to understand the information and the behavior and asking for and granting forgiveness, which may enable moving out of a stuck position in the relationship.

In cases where confidential information from an individual session is agreed to be more potentially hurtful if shared than the feeling of betrayal at not having been let in on everything, the couple understands that sharing painful information, as well as withholding that information, has its price. Some people may not be able to continue a relationship with secrets. Others may be able to move forward in the present, knowing there is confidential information not known, respecting the other's judgment that not knowing may be more respectful than burdening the other. This is very controversial territory. Many clinicians state that they won't proceed with a couple where there are family secrets. Complete openness, or nearly so, while an ideal in good, caring relationships, may not be feasible in relationships with high conflict, an impasse, or a breakdown. Rather than setting absolute rules for dealing with secrets or confidential information, coming as close as possible to absolute disclosure or sharing—without creating worse problems of devastation, loss of self-esteem or positive self- regard—may be a wise course of action.

Before the end of the first session, each member of a couple is given the "essential list" (rational structure number five). This list, known colloquially as the "list in black and fright," indicates that each of them is a unique individual, expected to have individual needs as well as strengths and areas of difficulty.

The Essential Lists

Before the end of the first session each member of a couple is given the following list of questions (rational structure number five). Each person's written answers to the following questions form what I call the essential lists:

1. What do you know you want and need in any good long-term relationship?

2. What do you know you cannot tolerate in any good long-term relationship?

3. What do you bring as problems/difficulties to any good long-term relationship?

4. What do you bring as strengths to any good long-term relationship?

I hand each person a copy of these questions and request that they individually write up a list based on these questions, and that they bring their lists to the second session. (Rarely does anyone not bring in a list to session two.)

Asking each member of a couple to create his or her own list indicates that each of them is a unique individual, expected to have individual needs as well as strengths and areas of difficulty. The lists also convey that individuals may not want to tolerate certain things in a relationship. Longings, desires, and needs that may have never been given expression are cited as legitimate. Owning what they each contribute as problems to any relationship helps individuals take more responsibility for themselves and blame one another less. Acknowledging their own strengths helps people at a time of crisis maintain a balanced view of themselves.

Most of the time the lists are not a litmus test of the relationship's viability, but occasionally they are. One woman newspaper reporter needed her husband to read about and discuss current events

regularly, especially those found in the *Washington Post*. Her husband, an artist,

needed her to be minimally knowledgeable about work in his medium. He never

read any newspaper, and she was studiously unaware of any contemporary art, let

alone art being produced in his medium. Their needs, under the wants and needs

column in the lists, indicated mutually exclusive needs and behaviors, which the

couple recognized instantaneously.

Some people object to list making, saying that falling in love is chemistry,

kismet (fate), and that one cannot quantify relationships.

Knowing one has a deliberate choice in selecting a life's partner seems just as

important as chemistry. Listing needs of individuals in a good long-term

relationship may point to problems that may well be at the interface between a

couple— with neither of them at fault or deficient. The lists point out to individuals their own legitimate needs, as opposed to the deficiencies in their partners. The mediation therapist needs to explain that the point of departure for the lists is the ideal situation for the individual and not the deficiencies of the partner, although those are inevitably factored in.

The experience of reading through the lists is like simultaneously running two videotapes of two separate individuals. Each film gives maximum exposure to each person, sparing the couple a demonstration of their interaction and how they have collided with one another. If after extensive individual sharing, a couple deliberately decides to live together, then the film we see is double-billed, starring not one but both partners.

Summary

In this shaping of the process stage, a contract between the couple/ family and the mediation therapist will be struck. The number of sessions and their frequency will be determined. You

85

will double-check to make sure that each partner understands the importance of acknowledging to the other that he or she has understood what the other is saying and even feeling, even when the first partner disagrees with what is being said. This acknowledgment principle is basic and needs to be internally understood by each member of the couple. You need to share with the couple your responsibility to them to be neutral and symmetrical in order to help them achieve balance between every member of the family. Your responsibility to be neutral and theirs to listen and acknowledge are important aspects of the contract between you and the couple or family.

By the end of a preliminary mediation therapy session, most couples and their mediation therapists will know whether the decision-making process is applicable for them. If it is, they will have made an implicit mediation therapy agreement providing the parameters for their work together with you during the course of the eleven or so sessions to follow.

[1] Haley, *Problem-Solving Therapy*, 174.

[2] Belenky, et al., Women's Ways of Knowing, 138.

[3] Haley, 172.

The Beneficent Overall Structure of

Mediation Therapy

I knew everything he was telling me. I remarked that I did not really need anything explained, and he said that explanations were never wasted, because they were imprinted in us for immediate or later use or to help prepare our way to reaching silent knowledge. — Carlos Castenada, *The Power of Silence*[1]

Advantages of a Structured Approach

Permeating the entire mediation therapy process are values, attitudes, and strategies that provide a *beneficent structure* for couples and families in crisis. This overarching beneficent structure provides a strong, caring, neutral holding environment for two people who are at serious odds with one another. For the mediation therapist, "being with" the couple or family means being fully present with the agonies and the ambitions of *each* member of the family.

The mediation therapist has faith in the structure and conveys this faith to the couple. In the course of twelve sessions she or he has many times seen a blend of strong emotion, rational stepping back, plus instruction in assertiveness, communication, negotiation, and decision making lead to individuals' knowing their own decisions and to their making a mutual or mutually understood decision. The mediation therapist informs the couple that *many* others before them have positively achieved their decision-making goals in mediation therapy. She or he indicates that the mutual nature of making life-changing decisions lessens the assumed guilt or responsibility that one person adopts when making a decision of this magnitude alone and imposing it on a partner.

As mentioned previously, mediation therapy is used for many types of decisions between family members, with divorce decisions only one type. In eighteen years of experience with divorcing families, my observation has been that unilateral decisions to divorce set the stage for ongoing intense feelings of rejection, rage, jealousy, and inadequacy. Because I know that unilateral decisions to separate lead—in the short and over the long run—to such intense feelings, I encourage people in mediation therapy to make mutual decisions, or at the very least mutually understood decisions.

Building upon the possibility for mutuality in the decisionmaking process, the beneficent structure of mediation therapy supports the tolerance of ambiguity about the future direction of the relationship. The mediation therapist conveys a positive value in a wait-to-see attitude. Not knowingness may be positively defined as the pursuit of the best possible future.

Because the couple senses they will be well guided in their search for their future direction, a feeling of safety and solidity in the structure is conveyed. The mediation therapist makes abundantly clear that the intervention will be balanced between the discharge of very intense feelings and rational problem solving. Through illustration, the mediation therapist conveys that there will be consistency in mediation therapy; she or he will always set limits on their fighting, will redirect nonproductive discussions or arguments, and will ask questions to set them thinking. She or he consistently conveys confidence in their own abilities to reach decisions and conclusions. The mediation therapist lets both individuals know that she or he is for them, supports them, and is advocating for the best decision for each of them. When one of them subtly indicates that unless the mediation therapist is *for* him or her and *against* the other, the mediation therapist takes the time to explain his or her loyalty to their unit: loyalty to their making the best possible decision for each and for both of them together. If one of the individuals cannot tolerate sharing the clinician with the partner, or is distinctly in opposition to sharing one clinician, a thoughtful referral should be made to separate psychotherapists.

Another aspect of the mediation therapy that conveys safety to the couple is that the mediation therapist will have explored his or her own biases about marriage and divorce and other relationships in order to learn to be neutral, but not valueless, about the outcome of relationships. Examination of the mediation therapist's biases about marriage and other relationships may be done by asking oneself specific questions, such as was undertaken in chapter 2 with the use of bias sorters. Alongside understanding one's own biases, the beginning mediation therapist is encouraged to incorporate the understanding, the *belief*, that people often have two very different, even oppositional, antagonistic positions that are *both true*.

In order to stay out of other people's polarizations, out of their either/or thinking, mediation therapists must be able to think in terms of grays, blends, effective mutual compromises, and nuances. They must be able to phrase their own disagreements as "I agree with part of what you are saying, but where I take a different view is on . . ." and, in order to model effective disagreement, they must have phased out polarizing statements such as "You're wrong!" or "I disagree." Open-ended questioning such as "How did that impact on you?" rather than "You must have been

hurt!" helps to preserve the neutral stance needed for a beneficent overall structure.

One of the basic conflict negotiation principles mentioned in chapter 6 is

funneling information through the mediation therapist. If, at the outset of the initial

session, the mediation therapist never allows a couple to display their fighting and

miscommunication, safety in the structure is conveyed. Paraphrasing what one

person is attempting to say, but without the negative body language, the toxic tones,

and gestures helps to disengage the couple from the helplessness that they must be

feeling in their inability to communicate. The mediation therapist must believe

that setting the rules, the limits, or boundaries in mediation therapy is his or her

province. The initial experience in mediation therapy must be different from what the

couple or family has previously experienced. The saving grace of the process is in

abiding by fundamental rules, the routines of the mediation therapy. Each couple's

story

unfolds within the structure of mediation therapy, which provides protection from the chaotic nature of their crises—for them, as well as for you, the mediation therapist.

Each couple's uniqueness quickly becomes evident in the structure of mediation therapy. Each couple brings a wealth of resources of its own to the process. Just as in a caring family, with clearly designated boundaries, each child may develop uniquely, without frequently having to test the boundaries and rules, so too in mediation therapy couples may, in a climate of safety, devote their energies to discovering their decisions about the future direction of their relationships.

As previously mentioned, the development of a neutral stance to structure mediation therapy does not mean the mediation therapist is morally neutral with regard to marriage or sustained long-term relationships. Valuing marriage, advocating the preservation of unions in which people grow emotionally, mentally, spiritually, and in which they may nurture any offspring in those ways, is not incompatible with being an objective neutral guide

for people to assess their relationship thoroughly.

An overall beneficent structure is conceptually oriented to provide limits

and boundaries within which couples have the autonomy to be guided in making their

own decisions. It is a safe structure within which toxic, really poisonous feelings may

be released. It is a structure in which couples may step back to see what has happened

and one within which they may get moving out of the stasis that has kept them

immobile and ensnared.

The overall structure of mediation therapy is one in which the mediation

therapist is sophisticated in guiding individuals to their own decisions, while

remaining neutral as to the outcome of the decision making. To a large degree the

mediation therapist controls the decision-making process, while the couple controls

the outcome of the process—their decision.

The Rational Structures

The rational structures are questions that are answered by the couple. Like several excellent photographs of an individual, they are revealing, but freeze several moods at specific points in time rather than conveying the essence of the person. Structures, like photographs, are only temporal evidence, frozen in time, of an ongoing process. To quote Castenada, "They are only one island in an endless sea of islands."[2]

—

My rational structures were named before Carlos Castenada's "flimsy rational structures" became known to me.[3] Adding the qualifier flimsy to my own rational structures does what I am trying to do in emphasizing that rational exploration, rational stepping back, while an important part of the decision making in mediation therapy, is but *one* aspect of an integrated process. Having stated that reason, emotion, and perception— seeing, hearing, feeling, intuiting, trusting, instructing— will be

96

equal guests in my intervention, I may introduce the rational structures of mediation therapy as "flimsy rational structures," good structural inquiries, which are not intended to stand on their own for decision making. After all, rational structures are questions *in words.* Inner knowing, the experience of leaping with courage to a decision, does not have words, initially: rather it is an *experience* of conviction, of intellectual, emotional, and sensory coming together with solidity. Once we know, we can look back at the rational structures to understand how and why we know what we know.

Rational structures are guided inquiries into the natures of the mediation therapy clients, into their relationship to one another and into their past and present situations.

Promoting rational self-reflection is the goal of the flimsy rational structures. Typically the structures are woven into the couple's ongoing dialogue with one another. For couples trying to make a marriage, or live-together, or go-their-own-ways decision, the twenty rational structures may often be posed to a couple consecutively, which is how the first several and last several structures are typically presented to couples. The middle structures are more interchangeable. There is room for modification, subtraction and addition to the rational inquiries. By themselves, the rational structures only go so far toward the attainment of silent knowledge or inner knowing.

The rational structures in mediation therapy will be described in detail in chapter 4. These rational inquiries are attempts to get couples to uncover and share what they know about themselves, as individuals and as a unit. The self-reflective process is intended to contribute to what Carlos Castenada might agree we could call the world of "silent knowledge" or what I call inner knowledge.[4] The rational structures stem from a need to get to a place of inner knowing.

—

Through a process of rational stepping back to observe themselves as individuals, and as a unit, and by expressing deep emotion between them, and within themselves, the individuals arrive at a place of deep inner knowledge of the direction they want to take in their futures. The rational structures allow them to travel backward from inner knowledge, through what Castenada calls "concern" to a rational understanding of how they know what they know.[5] People's logic, their linear thinking, will be satisfied, in that not only will they know a decision, but they will now be able to explain *how* they know— to themselves and to significant others.

Other Strategies

The rational structures coexist in mediation therapy with uncovering the perceptual channels—visual, auditory, kinesthetic—that were previously blocked and distorted. The perceptual channels become islands of seeing what is really there, and of hearing what has been said and not said, and of feeling what one honestly feels. The safety of the structure in mediation therapy, additionally, encourages and allows the sharing of emotions at such depth that long-standing emotional blockages to understanding are frequently cleared, creating passageways of understanding between people. A man in his forties sobbed deeply remembering his dog, Patches, who was taken away when he and his mother had to move from their home, when his father went to prison when he was seven years old; his wife sat by, tears rolling down her cheeks. Another woman sobbed about how stupid she still feels as a result of her mother's criticism of her.

People in mediation therapy are given instruction, often for the first time in their lives, in the art and science of assertiveness, communication, negotiation, and decision making. They are encouraged to become aware of their intuition and of their own inner wisdom. The process of decision making in mediation therapy is not a linear, solely rational process, but encompasses the person using every avenue of understanding, including the cognitive, that he or she has at her disposal.

A confluence of many kinds of information—sensory, educational, emotional—not just rational, contributes eventually to decisions that are experienced with a sense of inner knowing. The twenty rational structures presented in the next chapter are genuine suggestions that will need to be modified to meet the unique needs of a specific decision-making population. There is instruction with each rational structure, but no instruction on when in the mediation therapy to present it for use with a particular couple, although as mentioned before, appendix A does offer one possible twelve-session plan.

Notes

[1] Castenada, *The Power of Silence*, 218.

[2] Ibid., 261.

[3] Ibid., 247.

[4] Ibid., 218.

[5] Ibid., 261.

The Rational Structures

Just like you, I trusted my mind, implicitly. The momentum of the daily world carried me, and I kept acting like an average man. I held on desperately to my flimsy rational structures. Don't you do the same.

—Carlos Castenada, *The Power of Silence[1]*

Rational structures in mediation therapy are designed to assist clients to see more clearly. Seeing more clearly, understanding themselves and their relationship more fully are the goals of the rational structures. The rational structures are interwoven with the educational and sensory structures, discussed in chapter 5. As stated in the last chapter, frequently the first three rational structures may be posed to a couple or family sequentially, and the last four or five structures may also be posed in order. The structures in between are usually varied in placement, determined by the mediation therapist's sensitivity to appropriate timing and placement of the inquiries. I list here the twenty rational structures that promote clearer seeing and cognitive understanding:

1. What are each individual's separate goals for the intervention?

2. What are each individual's theories about the breakdown or impasse in the relationship?

3. How does each individual think their family of origin (FOO) or other significant parenting figures, would view their relationship crisis if they knew everything that the individual knows about it?

4. The impertinent questions: What attracted each person most to the other? What does each person like most about the other? What bothers each person most about the other? What would each person miss most about the other if the couple should ever separate? Trace major fights, themes of the fights, and so forth.

5. The essential lists.

6. What main internal issue is each person dealing with right now?

7. How do the first several years, or months, of the

        relationship compare to the last several years or months?   Were

there identifiable stages in between?

8. What positives have there been in the relationship?

        Which remain today?

9. What negatives have there been in the relationship?

        Which remain today?

10. What are the repetitive patterns in the relationship?

        The poulet-oeuf (chicken-or-the-egg) questions?

11. What are the collective issues in the relationship?

        Which aches, gripes, conflicts, and anxieties would need   to   be

resolved for the couple to have a rewarding relationship?

12. The geneogram depicting how the individuals'

        extended families have handled conflict.

13. Instruction in the importance of mutually understood,

        if not mutually agreed-upon, decisions.

14. Clarification of past misunderstandings and asking of

forgiveness.

15. What will individuals carry forward into the future, whether living together or not?

16. An emotional sharing from the heart and a rational listing of alternative future directions.

17. Individual decisions reported, and negotiation to mutual or mutually understood decision.

18. A negotiated settlement between the two individual decisions.

19. Information about children's needs during crisis.

20. Planning the next steps after the negotiated settlement.

Rational Structure Number One:
Each Individual's Goals for the Intervention

This structure always occurs in the mediation agreement phase of the process, and it serves to separate the individuals out from the problems between them. Beginning the intervention by stating one's own goals for the intervention is a far cry from: "He or she *always* or *never* does X, so that I never get Y!" The mediation therapist's request to the individuals to state their goals helps individuate each individual, empowers each to view the potential effectiveness of the intervention as being within his or her own control and gives him or her a positive future-orientation. The request for goals makes it impossible to begin the intervention with character analysis and defamation, blaming each other, or with a focus on the past.

The initial focus is on the future, on what the individuals want in their lives. There is a deliberate defocusing from what went wrong, from blaming and accusing. Sustaining this positive frame of reference is critical for the progression of this decisionmaking intervention. Respect is paid to the importance of the partnership, while, at the same time, the initial focus is on each individual who makes a separate, personal statement. The process is begun with a direct and emotionally unladen sharing of individual needs and desires.

Rational Structure Number Two:

Each Individual's Theories about the Impasse

Rarely do individuals view the breakdown or impasse in their relationship in exactly the same way. Openly expressing how each partner views what contributed to the difficulties has the possibility of broadening an individual's overly simplistic understanding of the crisis in the partnership. The focus of people's theories is often less on finding fault and more on specifics: communication, sex, money, children, in-laws, being two entirely different types of people. Indeed, at least in heterosexual couples, the members of the couple are more different as a man and a woman than they have come to view themselves in their recent search for equality. Many couples have mistaken equality for sameness. She expects him to be as satisfied with listening and talking as he expects her to find rewards in quiet togetherness and mutual participation in activity.

Each partner hears the other's theories and priorities. There is no other possibility than to compare and contrast how each one views the crisis. The mediation therapist takes the time to be certain that each individual has heard and *understands* the other's theory about the impasse.

Each rational structure conveys a message alongside the question it poses of the partners. The "medium," or the form of the question, may well be the most important part of the message. In this case the fact that the question is asked conveys the following message: you are separate people entitled to view your crisis from your own individual standpoint. That the mediation therapist is recognizing and acknowledging each person's individuality and way of seeing the world is as important as obtaining each person's theory.

Rational Structure Number Three: Family of Origin's
Point of View

Assume your family of origin (FOO)—that is, your parents or other significant parenting figures—know everything you do about the crisis in your relationship. What do you think they individually would think about it? This question challenges individuals to put themselves in their parents' place, to think as their parents have come to be known to think. Secondly, it gives the individual the opportunity to know that this viewpoint is, indeed, the viewpoint of the parent, not necessarily one's own viewpoint. Or, the parental viewpoint may indeed be one's own internalized parental message or superego.

A clear example of the former is Mary, a woman who stated that her mother's view most certainly would be extremely negative about her daughter divorcing, due to her orthodox religious views. Mary, herself, had been feeling very burdened by her decision to divorce, but realized that she views divorce considerably more liberally than her mother. Mary had been assigning more weight to her mother's strict orthodox views than to her own. When she differentiated her own values from her mother's, she became freer to empathize with the impact her decision was having on her mother.

This *circular question*—asking a question about another's viewpoint—is an indirect route to the individual's knowing how he or she views the relationship crisis. Answers to how one's family views one's crisis are frequently multifaceted: "My mother would like to see us work on our relationship for the sake of her grandchildren, but my father never did think the marriage would work and is probably saying 'I told you so.'"

This question gets at introjects, internalizations, the superego. It can separate out the involved person's own conscious viewpoint from preconscious and unconscious internalizations. The answers may help the client, as well as the mediation therapist, to assess how differentiated a person is from his or her parents.

Thinking about how another views one's own situation tends to prompt one to clarify how one views the situation oneself.

In mediation therapy, delving into family patterns in order to change maladaptive patterning is not a central goal. So it is that some of questions, which would be pertinent in family therapy, may seem impertinent in a decision-making process. Mediation therapists ask the following questions randomly, when appropriate, to increase clients' understanding of themselves and of each other for the future, in or out of the relationship:

1. What attracted you to your partner (your mate, your
    spouse) in the first place?

2. What do you presently like the most about your
    partner?

3. What did your partner bring to your unit that you
    lacked at the time you got together? Which of these characteristics
still -contrast with your own characteristics?

112

4. What would you miss most about your partner if the
     two of you should ever decide to part?

5. What presently bothers you the most about your
     partner?

6. What do you presently need, want, or count on from
     your mate that you could and would like to do for yourself?

7. Do you see yourselves as being similar, as true
     opposites to one another, or just on opposite ends of the same
continuum (that is, both having
     trouble with control, but partner one being overly neat and partner
two overly messy)?

8. Are the difficulties between you recent and acute or are
     they long-standing? Are they a threat to the relationship?

9. What fears, if any, do you have about being alone or not
     in the relationship should you part?

10. Trace your major fights. What were the overt and the
     underlying causes?

11. What skills do you still desire to learn from your
partner?

12. What are the factors that tie you together?

These questions, for the most part, were devised by Priscilla Bonney Smith, a student of mediation therapy.[2] They help a couple identify for themselves whether they are more complementary or opposite, or whether they are more symmetrical or similar. The questions help the couple to begin to assess what they may have wanted to make up for, in themselves, in their choices of mates. They begin to indicate to the individuals how independent and separate they are or how merged together and dependent they may be. The impertinent questions, ideally, help a couple tolerate the examination of how they might cope, should they desire or need to separate, to live apart, or how they might cope if they decide to live together.

The third question—What did your partner bring to your unit that you lacked?—gets at the positive side of what the individual undoubtedly now considers a very detrimental trait. It is my conjecture

that when a partner is perceiving this trait negatively it is often because he or she is

feeling a dire deficit in him or herself of that quality that was originally lacking and

that helped to draw him or her to the partner.

Occasionally, the mediation therapist may want to present a couple with the

whole series of questions, in an attempt to help
them   view   their   asymmetry/symmetry,

independence/dependence. Couples who are attempting to make marriage

decisions are most appropriate for this serial inquiry. However, more typical than

presenting the list of questions, these impertinent questions are part of a mediation

therapist's basic knowledge and are asked when they are pertinent to the

therapeutic discussion.

As with all the rational structures, these impertinent questions are meant to

increase peoples' perspective of themselves and of their relationship(s) and to help

them begin to

accept what they see. The questions may also help the couple focus on the fact that their relationship, like every relationship, has a positive and a negative aspect; they need to appreciate that there is always a little bit of good in the worst relationships, and a little bad in the best relationships.

It should be apparent from some of the answers whether or not individuals enhance each other's strengths and whether or not a partner originally attempted to fill in gaps or missing qualities in him or herself in the choice of a mate. Some people may choose partners who are at the far end of a spectrum upon which they simply desire to be located; they wish to be more orderly, but have chosen someone so impeccable that there is no comfort in living with him or her. With the impertinent questions it may be apparent that their similarities are stultifying or that these similarities reinforce positive aspects of a person.

These questions may highlight the positive aspects or the

oppressive aspects of complementarity or symmetry. They may help people to once again develop a sense of appreciation of themselves. Again, as with the other rational structures, the questions alone, even without the answers, are messages. Information, creepingly, helps people build a foundation on which a decision will rest. The impertinent questions, like the essential lists that follow, may be given to couples or families to complete at home to bring to a later session for discussion.

The point of departure of all of the impertinent questions is the individual self. Since couple decisions are composed of individual decisions, which are negotiated, the individuals in crisis in their relationship gravely need more information with which they may begin to arrive at an inner knowing of the direction to take with their relationship. The impertinent questions are designed to help the couple see more clearly, in order that they may eventually know more deeply.

Rational Structure Number Five:

During the initial mediation therapy session, a couple will be given the following list of questions. As mentioned before, a few individuals object to list making, saying in essence, "I couldn't possibly quantify these very personal, emotional aspects of myself into a list. You don't write your feelings down, you have them." Surprisingly, however, the great majority of individuals happily complete the task, rarely forgetting to return to the second session without lists in hand. In my experience, this is a decidedly greater return than for most homework given in psychotherapy.

The Essential List

1. What do you know you want and need in any good long-term relationship?

2. What do you know you cannot tolerate in any good long-term relationship?

3. What do you bring as problems/difficulties to any good

long-term relationship?

4. What do you bring as strengths to any good long-term
relationship?

During session two, individuals are instructed to keep their lists in hand and are asked, alternately, to read them aloud. Breaking the reading into eight parts with both people alternately reading answers to each question, then giving reactions to each other's answers (including sharing how many of the qualities listed under that question are present in their relationship), is a suggested point of departure. This breakdown of questions allows people to respond immediately to what they have just heard. If they don't spontaneously respond to each other's lists, the mediation therapist asks them, broadly, what their response is to what they've just heard. Sometimes people are bewildered by a partner's response, sometimes pleasantly surprised, reinforced, or challenged. Often people compare and contrast their responses saying, "We want the same things; why don't we get along?" or, "Of course we don't get along!" Often enough, individuals spontaneously comment that people with their particular individual problems will naturally have difficult times with one another. They see the coexistence of their separate, but negatively interlocking problems, as problematic for the unit.

If their individual problems/difficulties overlap in an obviously destructive way that the individuals do not mention, the mediation therapist may diplomatically draw attention to the overlap. She or he may indicate that in some problematic relationships individuals have wants and needs or "cannot tolerates" that are not compatible. Then the problems lie at the interface between the two individuals, rather than within one or the other of them. Rather than being people with incorrigible personalities who are intransigent to change, it is possible that there may be two idiosyncratic individuals with their share of difficulties, and also with incompatible needs. In other words, it is not necessary to see every partnership that does not work as someone's fault. For example, very occasionally the lists have served as a litmus test determining whether or not a relationship would work. A former civil rights lawyer indicated on her needs list a mate who cares about discrimination. Her ornithologist husband indicated that he needed someone who is particularly appreciative of nature and birds. He had no passion whatsoever for civil rights and she, with her passion for people, had no time for birds. The occupations of both of these individuals were also their avocations. Although they respected one another, they decided there was not enough commonality in their lives to feel satisfaction in their partnership. The complementarity, rather than enriching their lives, left each partner feeling alone. This was apparent on their lists. She wrote: "I need someone who rather passionately or least moderately passionately cares about discrimination of the less fortunate and minority peoples." He wrote: "I cannot live with someone who doesn't know a robin from a wren."

More often, the essential lists are not litmus tests, but become worksheets. Areas of compatibility and difficulty are highlighted for future work or to serve as a current understanding of the excessive difficulty the couple is experiencing in making this relationship work.

In over ten years of practicing mediation therapy, some differences between what men and women want in a good longterm relationship have become apparent. Women typically describe wanting emotional closeness as meaning wanting talking and listening while men use the same words to mean a participatory sharing, doing things quietly or actively together. One man honestly described the seven hours he and his wife spent in bed each night as being emotionally close. His wife said that this would be close only if one of them, at least, were talking.

The essential lists put yearnings, limits, and core personal difficulties into words and visual representations. When these important personal requirements are merely alluded to, or barely spoken out loud, they may not be taken seriously, or even seen as legitimate. The lists may be frightening or evoke some resistance in a few people. These individuals may anticipate that they will recognize needs and desires that are very important for them to have in a relationship. At the same time, they fear they will recognize that there is very little hope of their realizing these desires in their current relationships.

It is natural for people to anticipate that these lists may lead to the conviction that action will be necessary. That action may be to see a need to improve themselves and their relationship. Or they may even acknowledge that further attempts to become effective, satisfied partners appear futile. Some other individuals may view achieving what they need and want in a relationship as selfish, and so object to making a list. A significant number of individuals may state the belief that people are wildly attracted to their chosen mates through chemistry or kismet. For these people, to rationally decide what one needs in another person or a relationship, is like trying to canoe upstream. Falling in love, without participation of consciousness, is a law of nature in this epistemology.

The question "What do you *know* you want and need in any good long-term relationship?" implies that self-reflection, learning from experience, choice, and rationality are equal, at the very least, to "falling in love," chemistry, and kismet. From the mediation therapy perspective, one falls in love, indeed with one's heart and emotions, but also with one's head and rationality, with one's eyes, ears, intuition, and inner wisdom— not simply as a product of chemistry. The lists proclaim this message to individuals: it is desirable to know yourself, what you want, what is healthy for you. It is not necessary to be entrapped by id, by unconsciousness, by chemistry, which is more than likely to be an attraction to the familiar.

The essential lists are written down and laid out for the individuals to see clearly. Making the lists involves the couple's stepping back from the heated contemporary situation into a position of individuated self-knowledge. The lists are about individuals, not about complicated interpersonal issues in which people may have merged their separate identities. Couples are told that in making the lists, the individual's point of departure might be that of a pristine young person with his or her future in front of him or her, combined with the perspective gained over the years in relationships and in life.

The lists are powerful because they force each individual to commit to words what he or she wants and does not want in a relationship. The lists provide a rational framework that makes into a conscious process looking for or evaluating a partner, challenging the notion of just falling in love. The lists enable individuals to step outside the relationship to view their relationship. They remove blame; what one likes the other may dislike intensely. This is a structural barrier rather than a personal deficit.

The lists are, in a way, "personalized depersonalizations," and they work to clarify what individuals want, because the individuals can literally see in front of them a visual representation of what they want and don't want, without blaming the partner.

Inevitably, what one does not want to tolerate in a relationship will be what has been gathered, at some expense, as information about oneself in the contemporary or a prior relationship. It is acceptable to list these gems of knowledge derived from past relationships. The point of departure for the lists, however, is not the current relationship, per se, but the individual self, including all of his or her experiences to date, not simply the negative aspects of the current relationship.

Rather than beginning the mediation therapy with the couple saying, in essence: "Here we are, we ran into each other, there was a gigantic collision and now we need to put the pieces together or call it a lost cause," we begin from a time perspective prior to the individuals' colliding with one another. We begin when they were still whole or, more likely, partially whole or partly formed individual entities.

Using this individual perspective in a "couple context" and controlled environment, mediation therapists figuratively project two video screens before them, one of each member of the couple. The partners appear separately, sounding wise from past experience. The individuals are aware of their needs and the difficulties each brings to a good long-term relationship. As they speak, the accompanying visuals of their experience move chronologically back and forth in time to depict the scenes from which they most likely gleaned their current self-wisdom. For example, one woman doesn't want to tolerate active alcoholism. The scenes of years of struggle with the disease, first with her father, then her husband, appear for her with her words.

Often people know their critical wants and needs because they have suffered from not having had these things; they also know what they cannot tolerate because they *have* experienced those things. Individual problems are often only visible as a result of people having been in relationships; these problems would not have come to light had people lived solitary existences. This is the positive aspect of experiencing problematic relationships.

Viewing the relationship from the perspective of the individual gives mediation therapists maximum exposure to seeing the actors in action. The usual perspective of the couple relationship at the onset of psychotherapy is one in which the couple automatically demonstrates how they have collided, their impasses and inabilities to communicate, their egregious pains and complaints. It is no small wonder that the psychotherapist often gets caught up immediately in the problems and miscommunications of the couple, which often enough present themselves simultaneously with the couple.

Using the essential lists, which have a distinctive individual perspective, gives the message that the individual came before the couple. The lists implicitly demonstrate the importance of setting limits, boundaries, and non-negotiable areas between individuals in a partnership. They encourage taking personal responsibility, rather than blaming or accusing the other. When one lists what one wants and needs in a good long-term relationship, one is stating what is unique about oneself, rather than demanding that the other be X way or provide Y attributes.

Indeed, in the lists, one is speaking about oneself and what one actually needs, not about the other's deficiencies or what the other cannot provide or give. The point of departure is listing legitimate needs of unique people, not preposterous needs or demanding items. The intention is that the individual be aware of the things he or she earnestly needs in a relationship, in order for it to be a good and long-lasting relationship. Adding asterisks, double stars or numbers to items on the list may help individuals weigh their criteria for good relationships and weigh the relative importance of those things they do not want to tolerate over the long haul. Later on, when assessing their alternatives for a future direction, they may see how their most important criteria for a relationship are or are not met by each of their alternatives for a future direction.

The implications of the second question of the essential lists —what one knows one cannot tolerate in a good long-term relationship—are many. First, it is legitimate, acceptable, and understood that one will not be able to tolerate certain behaviors, which, for the listing individual, are non-negotiable. Second, the message of the question is that a good relationship is not just "anything goes." Having leverage is legitimate. It means that each person has standards, expectations, limits, and boundaries that need to be met.

Finally, the statements of one's own problem areas and strengths regarding relationships carry the message that, in mediation therapy, responsibility is expected of each individual; that blaming and accusations are not only ineffective but, in this intervention, are actually outlawed. Concerns may be transformed into "I" statements, that is, "I feel diminished when you talk about my sloppiness," rather than "You always make me feel bad about myself." "I" statements mean being able to talk about one's own problems and strengths objectively. Before talk of the relationship and any of its difficulties begins, the lists enable people to take a good, solid look at themselves, separately.

A partner often may feel so grateful that his or her counterpart can acknowledge difficulties that it makes it easier to acknowledge his or her own foibles. The second person's feelings and stance toward the other may, by virtue of the acknowledgment, become more positive: "Even if my partner has this difficulty, at least he or she is aware of it and admits it openly."

Sometimes people become aware, through their mutual listings, that their interactional difficulties result from a poor fit between their problems, rather than just from the difficulties themselves. For example, if one partner knows that one of her major difficulties in relationships is being too confrontational with everyone, and her partner knows that he loathes confrontation to the extreme, then some of their difficulty obviously lies at the interface between them, not just within each of them.

If people cannot cite any of their own difficulties or problems, the mate often will say that this inability is a major problem; the other has blind spots about realizing contributions to the relationship's difficulties. Or the first person may state that living with a saint has major problems.

Rational Structure Number Six: Each Individual's Main Internal Issue

What main internal issue is each person dealing with right now? More often than not, individuals want specific examples of main internal issues. Some main internal issues have been:

finding a meaningful first, second, or third career

achieving autonomy in decision making from one's
parents, spouse, or boss

finding a secure identity as a parent, partner, or worker

preserving feelings of independence, while learning
interdependence in a relationship

handling one's own or one's parents' aging

dealing with an illness or handicap in oneself, a child, or
parent

struggling with one's sexual orientation dealing with

success and its aftermath

beginning to deal with one's rage at not having gotten
enough emotional supplies in childhood

grieving the loss of a person or place or capacity such as
fertility, agility, memory

dealing with the agony of the unknown possibility of
inheriting a dreaded genetic disease.

Each individual's acknowledging and taking responsibility

for his or her internal issues has an obvious impact on the relationship. Taking responsibility for one's own struggles makes it less likely that those issues will manifest as a disturbance of the relationship. Throughout the life cycle, individuals will continuously have personal issues to deal with; it is probably not realistic to expect to be ever finished with personal issues. It is, however, realistic to expect to receive support from significant others in dealing with painful personal issues, without needing to attribute the pain to the couple or the family.

The thrust of the questioning in this and the other rational structures points away from blaming and accusing the other and toward taking responsibility for one's self and one's own issues. Again, as elsewhere in the structures, the "medium" is the message: You have internal issues. What are they? They are yours and do not belong to the couple.

Rational Structure Number Seven:

How do the first several years, or months, of the relationship compare and contrast to the last several years or months? Were there identifiable stages in between?

These questions are intended to provoke a broad overview, not a detailed accounting. If seeds of discontent or inappropriateness have existed since the beginning of the partnership, they will surface here, as will nostalgic reminiscences of a better past. Comparisons to the present will be poignant, and stages in between may have been normal developmental stages or may represent a roller-coaster-like, progressively worsening situation.

I imagine that not many people unite in a relationship without at least thinking or believing that there are some positive reasons for doing so. While experience may have proven them in error, this question reminds them of their own positive and good, if naive, intentions.

If people remember elements of their original compact for togetherness; if they still reinforce each other in their life's work, even though their parenting styles have made them seem to be adversaries, this question may remind them of the goodness that appeared lost in the midst of their troubles.

However the relationship compares and contrasts with itself, the couple is advised to be aware of how their togetherness has stayed the same, changed, gotten better, and/or gotten worse. Have the individuals grown and matured during the time they have been together? Has the relationship grown and matured? Or have the individuals (and the relationship) stayed the same or gone backwards?

The use of charts depicting stages in the life of a couple seem to be appropriate for couples to use to gauge whether their difficulties seem to be in or out of line with

normal

developmental stages for a couple relationship. The chart I use to describe the stages of a couple relationship is found in Appendix D.

What positives have there been in the relationship? Which remain today? Paralleling the power of misunderstandings to hold a couple together is the power of positives to hold a relationship together. There is the hope that those positives will be enough to sustain a relationship over the long haul. Asking an individual whose relationship is clearly destructive to him or her about the positives in his or her relationship may, paradoxically, be the fastest way for him or her to see the destructiveness of the relationship. Since no relationship is all bad, helping an individual recall that although her vacations with her husband throughout the years were the highlight of the relationship, this was not enough to allow them to survive year-round, since one does not live by vacations alone. Not talking about the positives in a difficult

relationship keeps the pain, the negativity, and, ultimately, the grieving at bay.

Acknowledging with the couple that most couples who make decisions to part, as well

as those who decide to stay together, experience positives in their relationship,

indicates to them that only by degree does one have a negative relationship or a

positive relationship. Those who stay together have had and will continue to have

hurts in their relationship, and those who judiciously decide to separate will have had

many positives in their relationships.

Rational Structure Number Nine:
Negatives in the Relationship

What have been the negatives in the relationship? Which remain today? At this point

in the mediation therapy, eliciting the negatives in the relationship gives

acknowledgment to those hurts just mentioned. Implicitly or explicitly, the couple is

asked to look beyond the dynamics of the immediate hurts and presenting problems and to forgive in the interest of moving forward with their lives and their relationship. Robin Casarjian, author of *Forgiveness: A Bold Choice for a Peaceful Heart*, describes forgiveness as a decision or choice to see beyond the reactive judgments of the ego in order to see that another's insensitivity and negative behavior is an expression of fear. She indicates her belief that all fear, at the bottom line, is a call for help, acknowledgment, respect, and love. She stresses that forgiving someone doesn't imply that we condone inappropriate or hurtful behavior, that we hesitate to establish clear boundaries as to what is acceptable to us, or that we act in a particular way. Rather, forgiveness is a shift in perception. It is another way of looking at what has been done that allows us not to take another's fear-based and insensitive behavior so personally.

Anger often masks feelings of helplessness, disappointment, insecurity, and fear. Forgiveness allows us to see with greater clarity and insight the fear and pain that lie

beneath the anger

and resentment. To quote Casarjian:

> As we gain the clarity to not personally take offense because of another's fears and projections, we won't fall prey to feeling victimized. Taking offense in a deeply personal way is the ego's way of keeping the real issues in the dark. Forgiveness releases us from weaving complex scenarios of anger, guilt, blame and justification. Forgiveness challenges us to deal with the real issues, to see fear for what it is and to develop clarity, establish boundaries, take explicit action when it is called for—all the while keeping our hearts open in the process.[3]

Forgiveness allows us to respond rather than react. Not to forgive is to be imprisoned by the past, by old grievances that do not allow our lives to proceed with new business and with the potential for loving and caring in the moment.

Casarjian says that "regardless of your current relationship with the people who originally provoked your anger, if you continue to carry it around with you, it is important to realize that you are now responsible for holding onto it, or choosing to let it go."[4] She believes that unresolved anger eats away at individuals' self-esteem, negatively impacts physical health, and always inhibits goodwill.

Casarjian cites many potential secondary gains that people can get from holding onto resentment, some of which are listed below:

not feeling the feelings that may lie beneath the anger:
  sadness, fear, hurt, disappointment, guilt, and so forth

staying in agreement with others who are also resentful getting attention

staying distant from others

avoiding intimacy

avoiding responsibility for one's part in what is going on not risking other

ways of being
avoiding the truth

feeling "right" or self-righteous

maintaining the familiar feeling of anger or resentment retaining the feeling

of being a victim—evoking sympathy

I tell my mediation therapy clients that I agree with Casarjian that forgiveness is a practical strategy: that to forgive releases both the other and the self. They are advised to fully acknowledge their deep disappointments, their rages, their sadness, and anger, and then to let them go, to release them forever. Forgiveness is a very important part of the mediation therapy process.

By asking about the positives and the negatives of the relationship, asking that people learn to forgive the negatives and hurtful aspects of the relationship, the mediation therapist is conveying implicitly that she or he is not interested in having clients stay stuck in the past with what has hurt or not been accomplished. She or he is interested instead in having them move forward individually and collectively with their lives.

What are the repetitive patterns in the relationship? The poulet-oeuf
(chicken-or-the-egg) questions? What patterns in your relating have you discovered
over the years? How do you usually express anger, disappointment, or sadness with
one another? What are the boundaries you construct between yourselves and the
world?

Couples frequently find themselves engaged in repetitive, predictable
struggles with one another, which they feel helpless to break out of or to change. I
call these the poulet-oeuf questions: Which came first, my doing X to you, or your
doing Y to me? For example, each autumn, she castigates him for being unavailable to
help with the storm windows and putting away the summer furniture; each autumn
he moves deeper and deeper into more and more important projects at work.

Family systems therapists have emphasized that there is an

emotional process between two people, a sequence of events that is circular and not linear, as opposed to a cause and effect sequence of events. Each person's behavior has an impact on the other, but does not cause the other to behave in a certain way. If a sequence of interactions between a couple is punctuated at any given point, a circular loop may be traced to see what one event follows the next, but a linear line of explanation cannot be made.

For example, let us punctuate the aforementioned situation at the point of the wife's identifying the need to take in lawn furniture and put up storm windows. We cannot assume that her husband is getting deeply into his work at this time in order not to do the seasonal chores. He may always be overwhelmed at work in the fall. His wife may be asking him for help (instead of hiring help) because it is less threatening for her to say she needs help with the house, than to say she needs her husband emotionally and physically. Or her husband may create work projects when home projects loom large. We simply do not know. We do know, however, that this dance of arguments about storm windows and lawn furniture occurs predictably for this couple on or around September 15 every year.

If couples can identify their ritual fights or dances, they may be able to work backwards, attempting to understand the emotional underpinnings. They may be able to give up repetitive, frustrating behaviors that undermine their individual and collective self-esteem. When the wife in our example was able to identify that she needed her husband emotionally, even when his work was at a peak, the arguments over lawn furniture and storm windows ceased. They began eating together near his office, several nights a week, and she hired a high school student to take in the lawn furniture and a fix-it person to adjust the storm windows. On the other hand, the husband could have been the first to break up the repetitive ritual dance by attempting to problem-solve with his wife when he recognized that she obviously had an important need.

Couples frequently ask for examples of ritual dances. The

mediation therapist can easily give examples from professional and personal experience. A typical ritual dance around the expression of anger in a heterosexual relationship is that a man will be furious internally about his own feelings of inadequacy, something he has done or feels unable to do, but he feels unable to share these feelings for fear of exaggerating them and making them even bigger than they are. He is withdrawn, uncommunicative, "dead" to his partner. His partner, not understanding that he is furious with himself, interprets his quiet, internal inferno as being unexpressed fury at *her,* even as rejection. If she then steels herself to his deadness, herself projecting an air of aloofness, he will, of course, interpret her behavior as reinforcement of his inadequacy. Breaking into this pattern, helping to create new ways of dealing with angry feelings, comes only after the identification of the ritual dance.

Another example of a ritual dance involving the expression of sadness involves a woman who over many years has been deeply sad about her mother, who is chronically ill. Her partner is compassionate, very empathic, but also obligated to be disciplined in his profession. When the woman becomes sad she relies on her partner, who very often is there to listen to her, hold her, and to understand. On the occasions when his own work or his own family problems preoccupy him, this woman responds hysterically: he must be involved with another woman, although she knows he is not; or: he has quit loving her and that they should no longer be partners. This pattern is predictable and does not occur when she is disappointed or angry. Only when she is sad and he is not fully available to her does she become super-sensitive; the sadness turns into suspicion and a hysterical pattern within their relationship.

Again, identifying the pattern is essential to breaking into it to create new ways of obtaining emotional needs—in this case, comfort for sad feelings. The woman in this example used a cognitive understanding to stop herself each time she began to accuse her partner of having an affair and to look within for sad feelings she might be in need of sharing.

Habitual responses to conflict are endemic. He wants to go to the woods for vacation, she to the shore. He always says they should take separate vacations, she always says they should divorce. No one ever suggests the lake with woods beyond.

Just as couples tend to have repetitive ways of dealing with angry feelings, sad feelings, disappointment, and conflict, they also tend to have fixed boundaries between themselves and the rest of the world. Boundaries within and between a couple and the outside world are typically static. Extensively adapted from Jurg Willi in *Couples in Collusion,* figure 4-1 represents three typical boundary situations.[5]

—

Figure 4-1. Boundary Diagram

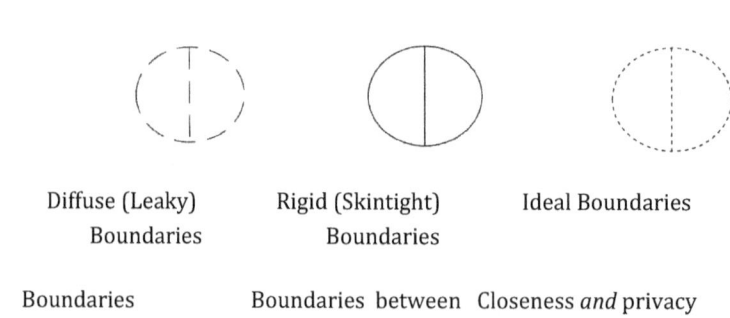

Diffuse (Leaky) Boundaries	Rigid (Skintight) Boundaries	Ideal Boundaries
Boundaries	Boundaries between	Closeness *and* privacy

between members of a couple and the world outside are too open, the sense of "we-ness" is not there. Boundary between the individuals is also too open; there is not enough privacy and separateness.	members of a couple and the world outside are too closed; there is stagnation for lack of stimulation, and connectedness to others. Boundary between individuals is too closed. Individuals are not intimate.	between members of a couple is preserved and there is connectedness to and distance from the world outside. Individuals preserve their privacy and independence, while joining in interdependence .

Source: Adapted from Willi, Couples in Collusion, 18.

The first diagram shows a couple with too-permeable boundaries between them

as individuals. They are "consorting to be schlepps" as one bright mediation

therapy couple described it; they are too close, too enmeshed in one another's lives.

In addition, the boundary between them and the rest of the world was too open; there

were too many people in their home at one time and they were out of their nest too

much of the time

to have a bounded sense of coupleness, a discrete sense of "us" as a unit. Their ritual patterns were over involvement in each other's personal affairs and neglect of their mutual needs as a couple.

The second diagram shows a couple with too rigid a boundary between them. Their activities and time are spent alone, separately; there is not enough of a sense of "we" as a unit. They do not, however, have the problems of enmeshment and collusion in each other's problems. This couple also has a rigid boundary between itself and the world outside. The individuals here don't let many people into their nonunit and seldom go out emotionally into the world of people. Their ritual patterns were under involvement with one another, as well as with the larger world. The final diagram illustrates an ideal couple admitting others to their partnership, preserving privacy for themselves and sharing openly with one another.

Structure number ten asks not that people solve their

repetitive, ritual patterns or dances, only that they identify some of them (not in itself

a simple task). In general, people do not fully enjoy being entrapped by their

repetitive patterns and do enjoy, to a degree, beginning to see what these patterns are.

If there is a chicken, will there always follow an egg? or was it the egg that creates the

chicken? If I push this button, will you always react in one predictable way? Is this our

ritual dance, with no real beginning and no real end? Sometimes this dance is a

repetition compulsion so strongly rooted in individual personalities that in order

to route out the tangled weeds, the whole bunch must be pulled traumatically out of

the ground—in these cases a dramatic separation of the partners in some way must

occur.

The entangled interaction may actually serve a variety of functions. For those who

genuinely fear intimacy, the ritual dance helps to avoid that kind of contact. For others

who would otherwise be totally isolated, the ritual dance may keep them connected

to another human being, however negatively.

151

Identifying the ritual dance or joint repetition compulsions is a beginning step toward assessing whether or not the behaviors must continue or not.

Rational Structure Number Eleven: Collective Issues

What are the collective issues in the relationship? Which aches, gripes, conflicts, and anxieties would need to be resolved for the couple to have a rewarding relationship?

This structure asks the couple to spell out those things that would have to be addressed and remedied for the couple to have a rewarding relationship. Matter-of-factly posing a long list of possible difficulties lets the couple know you expect there to be problems in any relationship, and that talking about them forthrightly is also expected. Yetta Bernard's "aches, gripes, conflicts, and anxieties" covers the ballpark of these feelings.[6] It doesn't take couples long to begin to answer this question, which may be posed several times by asking, "Have you forgotten

152

anything?"

At this juncture, problem solving is not necessary; the notso- simple description of the aches, gripes, conflicts, and anxieties is the point. Problem solving needs to come later. When couples try to move into a problem-solving mode at this stage (when they are supposed to be concentrating on identifying the problems between them), the mediation therapist gently but firmly sets limits on the discussion, separating identification of issues from the actual problem solving. (In-depth problem solving of collective issues could occur in a subsequent contract after the completion of mediation therapy.) Making a decision with good understanding of what the individual and collective issues are is ambitious enough for the mediation therapy contract. On the other hand, if couples *strongly* request that the mediation therapist help them work on and resolve a single issue, the request may at times be granted.

As was done previously with other questions, the couple is

asked whether these interpersonal issues pose a threat to the relationship (see

rational structure number four). People readily indicate in the affirmative if the issues

pose a threat to the relationship, even though they typically are not happy to see and

admit this threat. The question separates toxic differences from terminal differences

and indicates the areas in which the couple needs to work if they decide that they

want to continue the relationship.

Examples of aches, gripes, conflicts and anxieties are: "I feel that you

constantly try to plan and control my life." "I don't feel loved by you on a daily

basis."
    "I yearn for a close and loving sexual expression with my
        partner."

    "I will not be able to forget or to forgive your affair." "I've never felt

that you *really listen* to me."
"You make important decisions which effect me, without

me."

Prioritizing the collective issues from most to least difficult helps a couple see in what order they would want to address the issues, when an appropriate time arises to work on them.

Rational Structure Number Twelve:
The Geneogram

Not every couple requires a specific, focused period of time during which a three-generational family map, or *geneogram*, is composed. The majority of couples, however, learn an enormous amount about themselves and their families by doing the homework assignment of individually composing a threegenerational geneogram focusing especially on the quality of relationships in the family of origin. The mediation therapist either draws a basic geneogram to illustrate what is expected, or gives clients forms, such as the one in figure 4-2, with instructions on how to complete them.

Figure 4-2. A Sample Geneogram

Complete each shape as outlined below in the Mother's circle. To signify death, place an X in the shape. To illustrate feelings between individuals, use the following symbols:

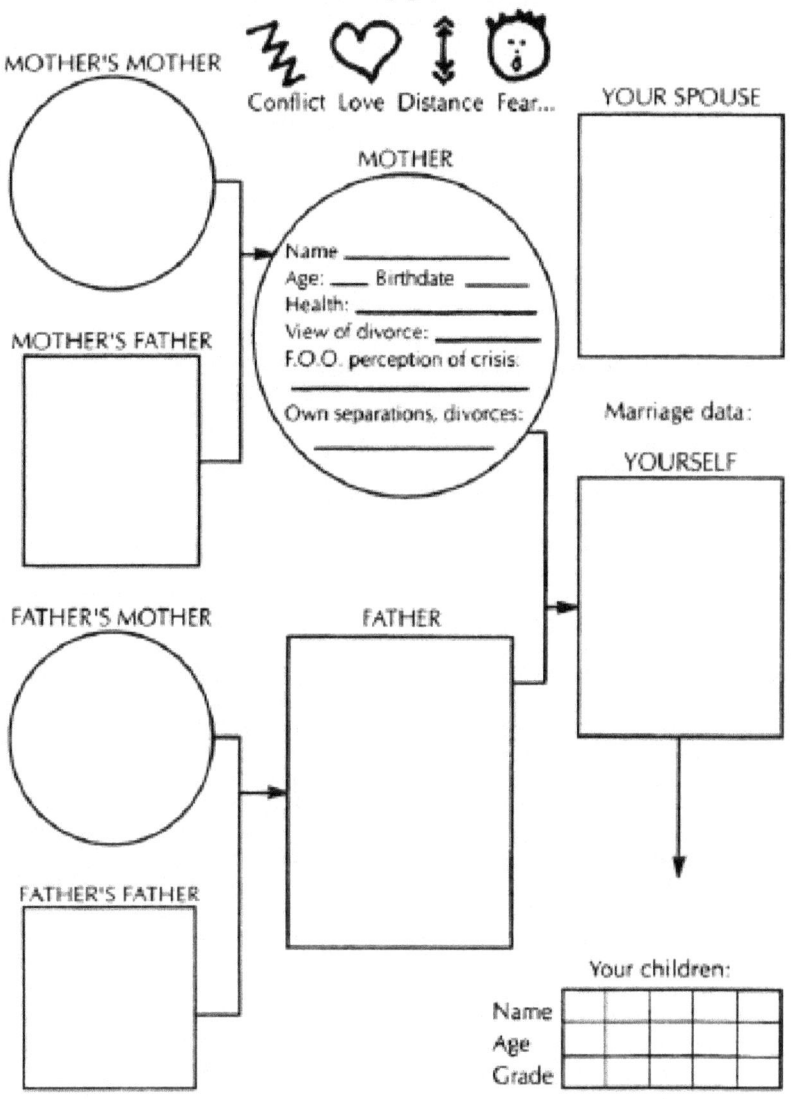

MOTHER'S MOTHER

Conflict Love Distance Fear...

YOUR SPOUSE

MOTHER

Name _____
Age: ____ Birthdate _____
Health: _____
View of divorce: _____
F.O.O. perception of crisis.
_____

Own separations, divorces:
_____

MOTHER'S FATHER

Marriage data:

YOURSELF

FATHER'S MOTHER

FATHER

FATHER'S FATHER

Your children:

Name				
Age				
Grade				

157

Source: Adapted by Janet Miller Wiseman, and Annette Kurtz, and Bob Wiseman from a concept by Murray Bowen.

Almost any information about each individual's threegenerational family system will be useful for the mediation therapist, but instructions are given to focus on the following:

5. How did couples in the family handle anger, sadness, conflict, and disappointment between them?

6. What are the attitudes of grandparents, parents, and yourselves about marriage, separation, divorce, and so forth.

7. Were there any models for good relationships in the family? Extended family? In the neighborhood? Anywhere?

8. List dates (and probable causes) of deaths, births, divorces, separations, anniversaries, adoptions, miscarriages.

9. List occupations, educations, interests.

10. Indicate medical, mental/biological illnesses, alcoholism, and so forth.

11. List any divorces, separations, living together without
    marriage, homosexual partners that you are aware of.

12. How did couples get along? Hearts (love), zig-zags
    (conflict)?

13. Add up the number of significant losses for you in your
    lifetime, through death, divorce, moves, and the like.

14. List areas of strength for all family members. Seeing a conglomerate of

losses may make it evident to

people why they cling to one another in the face of great conflict and tension between

them; they may feel they simply cannot endure another loss.

For the most part, couples in mediation therapy have enjoyed and learned from

making their family maps. Clearly the focus in doing this specialized geneogram is on

how couples have gotten along or not gotten along, what they have done to solve their

difficulties or how they have institutionalized them.

159

Sadly, individuals do not realize that, unwittingly, they are emulating the other models they have seen, trapped by the only visions they have seen for interaction in relationships.

The heat is taken off the couple relationship during the time they construct their family maps, because the maps remind them that they did not grow up in a vacuum, that they have a context for experiencing relationships. Before the contemporary problematic relationship were relationships that may have inadequately prepared them or negatively influenced them for being in a loving, intimate partnership. Especially important to individuals is to be reminded of how their models or antimodels handled conflict, which they are so totally immersed in at the moment. The intent is to help individuals achieve understanding and self-compassion, not rationalizations for difficult behavior.

Frequently the form for making the family map is given to couples at the end of the third or fourth session. If, for some reason, the mediation therapist does not have time

or thinks it

inadvisable to request a geneogram from the couple, she or he will want to make one

him or herself, including the information the individuals give about their perceptions

of their parents' views of their crisis (FOO perceptions) and their individual theories

about the breakdown in the relationship. The mediation therapist's geneogram will be

a shorthand visual notation of the individuals' family contexts, relationships, and

attitudes. Copies of the geneogram made by the mediation therapist or of the couples'

geneograms can be made for the couple and for the mediation therapist. Asking for

areas of strength, including beliefs, values, spiritual or religious orientation

makes the geneogram more rounded and less focused on problem areas.

Rational Structure Number Thirteen:
Importance of Mutuality in Decision Making

By about session six, the mediation therapist begins to offer instruction in the process

of decision making. While instruction in decision making will be elaborated in chapter

7, suffice it to

say here that explicit statements are made to the couple, approximately halfway into the process, that indicate the therapist's confidence in the couple's own decision-making abilities. She or he reminds them that thinking, reasoning, deducing are only part of the process—the head part.

As they have been gathering rational information about themselves, their families, and their relationships, the individuals have also been expressing what is in their hearts, that is, their emotional selves, to one another. They have also learned, symbolically, to take the veils from their eyes to see what is actually there in their relationship. They have taken the plugs out of their ears to hear what they are saying to one another. More important, they have learned to hear what they are saying to themselves. They have been instructed to listen carefully to their intuition—(what they know without thinking) and to their inner wisdom— what their guts, essences, and inner selves know.

The couple is reminded, in timely fashion (in a reinforcing, "hypnoticlike" suggestion), that they have been gathering sensory, rational, and emotional information and that they are, at this point, much better prepared than they were, initially, to leap from well-rounded information, with courage, to a decision, that place of silent knowledge or inner knowing. The suggestion that they are becoming more capable of making a decision appears to give people confidence in their abilities at this time to move into a decision-making mode.

Rational Structure Number Fourteen:

Clarification of Past Misunderstandings and Asking of Forgiveness

Having prepared the couple with the permission and encouragement to make decisions, or rather to recognize their decisions, the couple is preparing to let go of their ambivalence, their indecision, their relationship as they knew it, and possibly of one another. It is appropriate at this particular time, and not before, to ask each of them to think about what they have done, or the other has done, that they believe was misunderstood, was incompletely understood, or was otherwise unfinished business. Perhaps there was an affair, the motivations for which were never completely understood by one or both individuals, or perhaps one of them wanted very much to work on the relationship during a trial separation, while the other partner understood the separation to mean establishing autonomy and separate time and space.

Once misunderstandings in the relationship have been clarified, the mediation therapist asks the couple whether there are situations for which they would like to ask forgiveness, or anything for which they would like to offer forgiveness. These unfinished misunderstandings, like the positive aspects of a relationship, tend to hold a couple together. Hope seems to spring eternal that one day, one will be able to *make* the other understand and everything will be all right. Or, one clings to the hope of being proven right or being vindicated. One hopes to have the slate wiped clean by cleaning up the misunderstandings. The model of forgiveness designed by Robin Casarjian, which was discussed earlier in this chapter under the discussion of rational structure number nine, is the suggested model for helping couples learn to forgive after their misunderstandings are clarified.

If partners are waiting for clarification of a past misunderstanding, they can neither move forward together in a positive vein nor move apart. Usually forgiveness is not possible without clarification.

Rational Structure Number Fifteen:
What Will Individuals Carry Forward into the Future, Whether Living Together or Not?

This structure may appear to be a trick question calculated to force the hand of the individuals about their decision, before they are directly asked what they desire the future of the relationship to be. It is. It automatically gets the individuals to the heart of their vision of their relationship in the future. When, for example Maria Taylor hears, "What do I want to carry over into the future from our relationship whether together or apart?" she most likely will leap to her vision of the future first, then think of what she would like to carry over. She may think that she wants in the future always to have her husband's daily support for her career doing ceramics, which positions her in the future as quite probably still being engaged in the marital relationship with her husband. Or she may want to carry over into the future a positive parenting relationship with her husband, which may or may not imply continuing to live together.

The structure of the question is suggestive. There are many things in most relationships that could be left behind to mutual benefit. Identifying what is enhancing, what is supportive, and what is positive to carry forward into the future helps people visualize the future into which they would like to grow.

Rational Structure Number Sixteen:

Having clarified past misunderstandings and having asked for forgiveness, having reassessed the positives and the hurts of the relationship and established what they would like to carry over into the future, people are frequently disposed, at this juncture, to share their emotions honestly with one another:

"I want you to know that no matter what happens in our

relationship, I will never forget or quit appreciating what you did for me when I was first recovering from my depression."

"I want you to believe me when I tell you that I know how

much I hurt you when I had the second affair—you were heartbroken."

"Our children will always know and respect you as their

father, and not someone else I might be with, or marry in the future."

"I believe the rockiness in our relationship this past year

had a lot to do with our decision making about

whether to be married, and I don't believe we will always have a rocky relationship."

Sharing emotions openly with one another is an important part of being honest with themselves and the other person, an important part of making a decision about their futures. Whatever has been concealed, or held back, those difficult positive and negative areas are given permission to be shared:

"I want you to believe that my homosexuality is not a
        reflection of my view of your attractiveness as a woman, and, in my view, does not detract from the legitimacy of our children."

"Even if our baby looks like the man with whom you had
        the crazy affair, I will love 'our' child as my own, for the rest of my life."

At the end of the emotional sharing, the couple is encouraged to allow the open spirit of their mutual sharing to continue onward and inward toward the open recognition of their individual decisions about the future direction of the relationship. They are encouraged to enter that place of inner knowing of their decision, rationally understanding it after the decision is known. Individuals are encouraged to know what they know already and to acknowledge to themselves what they know.

If appropriate for an individual couple, at this point they are each asked to list alternatives for a future direction. A disenchanted but conservative wife might list as her three major alternatives:

· Postpone all decision making until all the children are
    out of college

· Separate for two years, then decide about the future of
    the marriage

· Separate indefinitely

Her unhappy husband might list his alternatives as:

· Divorce immediately

- Have wife move out of house, separate for two years,
  then decide

- Leave for Alaska next month

How each alternative matches what they want to accomplish in mediation therapy—to get out of limbo and become better parents—and matches what they want and want not to tolerate in a good long-term relationship is examined. Final decision making about the future direction of the relationship is specifically not attempted at this time.

Rational Structure Number Seventeen:

Individual Decisions and Negotiation to Mutual or Mutually Understood Decision

When individual decisions are called for, they are typically shared with great sighs of relief. They may have arrived at a decision earlier and shared it then, or waited until this point. Some few individuals will not have yet unearthed their decisions. If the individual decisions are the same—we each decide to stay married and build upon our foundation, or we each decide to separate, or divorce, to marry, to become engaged —there are only the conditions to be negotiated and children's or family's needs to be discussed. They may have decided to help his mother buy a multilevel medical care condominium, rather than building an addition to their home, but have the financial arrangements yet to agree upon.

Like genes, when individual decisions are disparate, one decision may be the dominant one, the other the recessive one, which is no longer seen in the final outcome. For example, a firm decision to separate or divorce will be dominant over a decision to stay together. How and when to accomplish the breaking apart are the issues left to negotiate. Nonetheless, helping the couple make the decision a mutually understood decision, if not a mutual or somewhat mutual decision, is, as was previously stated, an important part of the process.

The mediation therapist will help the person who wants the

relationship to continue, to accept and understand the hows and whys of the other's decision. More important, the mediation therapist needs to be able to help that person understand the destructive aspect of wanting to continue in a relationship with someone who clearly does not have the same goal—and his or her resistances to acknowledging this destructive aspect. Attempting to help that person fully understand the other's perspective and feelings contributes to a mutually understood decision.

Angry and vengeful feelings, and feeling rejected, are frequently present in a nonmutual decision and may propel a person to undertake the separation and divorce actions that otherwise he or she might be too paralyzed or depressed to undertake. It is not suggested that the mediation therapist attempt to modify the defense line of anger. The mediation therapist is encouraged to respect the angry feelings and to aid the partner at whom they are directed to accept that anger, without having to like it or agree with its causes. Understanding the perspective of a partner leaving a relationship does not entail liking the decision or curbing one's anger about the decision.

In chapter 6, techniques for negotiation and conflict resolution are comprehensively discussed. Some of those techniques are used here to help couples negotiate their individual decisions to mutual or mutually understood decisions. For example, if the members of a couple have both decided individually to separate, they will need to discuss the goals and the meaning of the separation, as well as its duration. Or, if one member of a couple knows definitively that she wants a divorce, while her husband believes in the potential of their relationship, what is not negotiable is the divorce, but what may be acceptable (in terms of negotiation) to the woman is an ongoing cooperative partnership around the parenting of their children. She is proposing divorce, and his counterproposal is the cooperative parenting partnership, which makes the divorce, not a mutual decision, but a moderately mutually accepted decision with the continued coparenting.

As much time as possible is spent at this stage of the mediation therapy so that individual decisions may, if possible, become mutually acceptable decisions to both members of the couple.

In the case of the couple with a decision to make about the location of his mother's home, he strongly felt that, out of loyalty to his mother, he should be able to provide a warm and congenial home, within his home. His wife strongly felt that her mother-in- law's steadily declining health, and her insistence on having daily meals cooked in old-world fashion, were reasons enough to want to have his mother at a geographic distance from the family, at a medical-care condominium. In this way she could easily receive medical care but live close enough to be a regular visitor to their home while she was able.

Her husband felt that his mother would prefer having her

own quarters within their home, and that it was his duty to provide this for her. When his mother's doctor shared his opinion that it would only be several years before the elder lady would require ongoing daily care, her son began a grieving process and accepted the preferability of the medical-care condominium for his mother. He negotiated with his wife the number of meals his mother could still cook in their home, and the number of visits each week that his wife and children would make to his mother at her condominium.

This couple described feeling good about the negotiation, which resulted in his mother living at a geographic distance from the home, where she could get medical care progressively as she needed, and still be a regular visitor to their home.

Couples are reminded that mutual decisions go a long way toward decreasing passion, abandonment, jealousy, and rage, currently as well as later, for the individuals and the couple. Individuals have the satisfaction of a mutually generated and created decision, which turns out often to be more optimal than either of their individual optimal positions. Mutual, mutually acceptable, or mutually understood decisions are experienced with relief. The individuals gain considerable energy, which was bound up in their indecision. Typically this decision making takes place in session ten, eleven, or twelve. At times, around session seven, as discussed previously, people ask for an extension of their twelve-session contract, so that there will be additional time for exploration and decision making.

More typically, around the latter two sessions, couples will ask what will happen if they don't reach decisions by the appointed time. I always assure them that they can have an extension if needed, but that I don't anticipate that this will be the case—that time is not infinitely on one's side in the decisionmaking process.

As mentioned in chapter 2, sometimes couples also want to know whether they may recontract for work after the decision making phase is over. As previously indicated, a break in time is recommended after a decision is made.

Rational Structure Number Eighteen:

Negotiated Settlement Between the Two Individual Decisions

The mediation therapist strives to help a couple or family achieve the highest level of understanding possible of each other's positions, for their own as well as any children's healthy adjustments in the future. If the understanding never comes, then the nonmutual position of their decisions is emphasized: "Anna Samuelson wants to go on the record as being in 'violent opposition' to the divorce, but as acquiescing to it, nonetheless." Putting positions on an imaginary record seems to go some way toward the person in opposition feeling that somewhere, someone has heard a profound opposition, that there is no complete understanding between them of why one partner has made the decision.

More typically, people will have both arrived at similar decisions, or they will have some understanding of why the partner has made the decision he or she has made. As stated previously, a dominant decision may obscure another decision, but there is typically room for negotiation about the timing of implementing a decision or about the conditions of the decision.

Rational Structure Number Nineteen:
Children's Needs

If, in mediation therapy, parents choose to divorce (or hospitalize a parent or child, or whatever), the mediation therapist may well dialogue with them about the needs of their children or their parents or others affected directly. Using the divorce example, research studies on effects of divorce on children, indicate that it is not primarily the structure of the living arrangement—either living with one parent, visiting the other, or living alternately with each parent—that determines children's adjustment; rather, a good adjustment results from high quality parenting over time and from parents considering their children a top priority.

I believe that at the time of divorce, each parent needs to take new vows of responsibility to the children, choosing where possible to take one hundred percent of the responsibility for all children, and choosing to learn new parenting skills. Many parents will need to learn to set consistent, firm limits with the children. Many others will need to learn to listen to their children, to nurture them, to be on duty constantly. It won't do to say to oneself, when the children are running wild: "Oh well, they have good limits at their other home"; or when they're hurt, "He [or she] cuddles them well when they're hurt." Complementary parenting will, of course, still be useful, but, when parenting alone, each parent will be called upon for a more rounded set of parenting skills than in a two-parent family.

Chapter 8 provides explicit information about children's needs at various age levels, boys' development versus girls' development, temperaments, and propensities to loyalty conflicts. Some parents will, advisedly, decide that their children need a network of extra support during the divorce such as seeing more of grandparents, aunts and uncles, beloved babysitters, or, in some cases, professional counselors. Accepting the reality that their parenting may well be diminished during the separation or divorce is a success rather than failure.

Rational Structure Number Twenty:
Planning the Next Steps after the Negotiated Settlement

Whatever decision a couple or family has made in mediation therapy, the individuals will soon need to begin to implement a plan for carrying out the decision. People who choose to divorce often discuss their children's needs and the mode of reaching their divorce settlement—usually negotiated through attorneys or a divorce mediator.

Couples who decide to live together decide when and in whose home, with what furniture and under what mutual agreements. Those who decide to marry often simultaneously rejoice and express

fears that the marriage may alter their relationship in frightening ways. Those who

stage a marriage or living together commitment over time heave a sigh of relief for a

moment that they haven't made a final commitment before they are ready, then with

the next breath a sigh of frustration that the ultimate decision still is not made.

Whatever decision a family or couple makes—joyously experienced or

with pain—they are out of the state of limbo, conflict, confusion, ambivalence. The

stress of not knowing, of being on the horns of a decision or dilemma, being stuck in

one position with no forward momentum, is over.

Summary

Combining the information gleaned from asking the above previously unrelated

twenty rational structures, yields a sum much larger than the individual structures.

This sum,

181

synthesized with the educational, sensory, and emotional structures is the integrated pool of information used by mediation therapy clients in their creative decision-making processes.

Notes

[1] Castaneda, The Power of Silence, 247.

[2] Smith, Priscilla Bonney, mediation therapy exam, Lesley College.

[3] Casarjian, Forgiveness: A Bold Choice for a Peaceful Heart.

[4] Ibid.

[5] Jurg Willi, *Couples in Collusion* (New York: Jason Aronson, 1989), 18.

[6] Bernard, "Conflict Resolution With a Couple," videotape.

Sensory and Instructional Structures

Most of the people I know are handicapped in terms of sensory ability. There is a tremendous amount of experience that goes right by them because they are operating out of something which is more intense than just "preconceived notions." They are operating out of their own internal world and trying to find out what matches it.

—Richard Bandler and John Grinder; *Frogs into Princes [1]*

You will always get answers to your questions insofar as you have the sensory apparatus to notice the responses. And rarely will the verbal or conscious part of the response be relevant.

—Richard Bandler and John Grinder, *Frogs into Princes [2]*

Our minds, devoid of collaborating evidence from the actual world, tend to spin their cognitive wheels. Our minds, without understanding from within and sensory information from without, remain in darkness.

Sensory Structures

How frequently do people enter a mediation therapist's

office, eyes squinted, brows strained, saying, "Oh, I am so confused; if I do X, I shall lose Y; if I do Y, I will certainly lose X. How will I ever know what I should do?" They are frequently surprised to hear the mediation therapist say something like: You are *thinking* too much. Open your eyes and ears to perceive, to observe what is really happening around you. You seem to be turning your eyes inward, viewing the conflicts going back and forth in your head. It appears to be an evenly matched tennis game, with you as the ball. You may decide it is time to give your mind a rest, to open your heart to experience your own true inner feelings and to be in contact with your intuition and your inner wisdom. You look as though you believe you *only* have a mind from which to receive information. Tune into the sound of your other fine senses. They will inform you at least as well as your mind.

As a mediation therapist, I take the view that sensory information is highly valuable. I agree with Joan Erikson, who said in *'Wisdom and the Senses,* "All that we

do have that is 184

genuinely our own is our personal, accrued store of sense data. That is what we really

know[3]." To quote further: "The sense information we have accrued through

experience is the most personal and valid content of our minds. What we store up in

our heads is the accumulation of experience made available to us through our senses.

All the other information we select and gather might legitimately be classed as

indirect knowledge based on what someone else has said or written[4]." Erikson

captures the point of congruency that one experiences when the senses and the mind

come together in solid understanding: "For the first time my mind and senses

collaborated and made the idea manifest. I understood. I knew[5]. "

—

It is this kind of integrated understanding that mediation therapists strive to help

clients achieve—an inner knowing that the decision that they have reached is the

right decision, even when it isn't what the person would want if he or she could

choose to control all circumstances. Adding sensory information to what the mind

knows may be a decisive factor enabling a

185

person to round a corner from confusion to inner knowledge. In *Women's Ways of Knowing,* Belenky et al. stated this concept well: [Women] are aware that reason is necessary, but they know, too , that it is insufficient, that to ignore the role of feeling in making judgments is to be guilty of something like 'romantic rationalism[6].'" What is needed is not reversion to sheer feeling but some sort of integration of feeling and thinking [and sensory information]. The authors talk about listening to a "voice of integration...that prompted her [a woman] to find a place for reason and intuition and the expertise of others[7]."

―

Verbal, conscious feedback is the stuff of the rational structures, described in chapter 4. If, as Bandler and Grinder say in the chapter epigraphs, we tap into the least informative part of the person with our rational queries and responses, we need to learn to tap into other parts of the person.

The sensory structures that concern this chapter are visual, auditory, kinesthetic, and intuitive; they ask people to tap into their own inner wisdom. Consciously, through being asked and answering the queries of the rational structures, people will have added a wealth of information about themselves. By acknowledging and opening up their senses, people will become more aware of what they know outside of their conscious minds. Not every person will be able to access all kinds of sensory information and need not be required to do so. A man who repeats that he is not a visual person, and does not see any image relating to the discussion, should be asked about what Bandler and Grinder call his predominant sensory "representational system":[8] "Which of your senses is most keen; touch, taste, sound, smell?"

—

I find it helpful to indicate to people my belief in the strength of their inner resources. I share with them my conviction that their knowledge, through their senses, is as important to them as their rational minds. "I believe that you have many inner resources for decision-making and can choose to be more aware of them than you have been to date" is the type of statement a mediation therapist may make to help an individual become aware of all that he or she knows on any level, to, as Brandler and Grinder put it, "induce impetus in the unconscious."[9]

—

Visualization

If at least one member of the couple has access to visual, metaphoric imagery, then the mediation therapist may ask that the quality of the relationship be visualized. For example, a mediation therapist might present a couple with the following sensory exercise: "Imagine you are together, opening a window on yourselves in the garden of your relationship. What do you see? Where are you sitting, working, lying, courting? What is growing there? How many weeds require uprooting? What is the general ambience—relaxed, stimulating, stagnating, desertlike? What little roots are underground just waiting to grow into the daylight?" In this metaphor, viewing the garden is taking an assessment of what is truly there in the relationship, as well as seeing what potential there is for growth. Mediation therapy requires the couple to own how they feel about being in the relationship, what constraints their togetherness puts on the individuals, as well as what spurs there are to growth.

As was stated earlier, sometimes people can acknowledge the reality of their relationship by putting it out in front of them, where they can see it more objectively than by simply using words. All the senses are brought into the picture by the use of the questions asked. People who cannot say that their relationship is floundering may be able to describe a garden that has become a silent desert of sumac trees or a bedroom in which there is no living thing. One woman described opening a door into her relationship. There she saw no people, only junk everywhere. Her husband described the relationship as a small picture that was clearly in the past. His wife appeared dressed in pink, svelte and self-assured. From this picture he commented that it appeared as if the relationship was in the past and that he had idealized his wife, refusing to see and accept her as she is now.

Seeing Clearly

From time to time individuals might be asked to remove any veils they have over their eyes in order to see clearly who they are, who the other is, what transpires within the relationship. A couple might be asked: "How much do you believe you distort how things actually are?" And if they do so a lot, does this *not seeing clearly* make aspects of their life appear to be more congruent, to be more whole, to make more sense? In other words, do they not see things clearly partially because to do so would be inconsistent with how they have told themselves things really are? If she doesn't see that he is spacing out most of the time, she won't have to acknowledge that his drug habit has probably recommenced.

Uptime is Bandler and Grinder's term for only being aware of sensory experience, and not of "internal feelings, pictures, voices, or anything else."[10] This is the opposite experience from creating a mental,

visual picture that describes the relationship. This uptime is consciously,

deliberately defocusing from all internal experiences to be aware of everything

around. Uptime in my view is seeing without judging, labeling, or distorting. Both

types of seeing, internal visualizing and external pure seeing, or uptime are helpful for

mediation therapy clients to know about. Visualizing the relationship can put it into

sharper focus for the visualizer and the partner. Seeing what really transpires in the

day-to-day world (not judging, labeling or distorting—just simply observing) may

open up untold revelations to individuals who have not been using information that

has been readily available to them: how thoughtlessly the partner behaves to

everyone, how the partner virtually never acknowledges what others say; how

agitated the partner has been about her or his work for some time.

Usually the mediation therapist will want to discern for her or himself when

it is appropriate for clients to attend to internal

cues, to internalizations or visualizations, and when it is most appropriate for individuals to tune out internal thoughts and feelings in order to be acutely aware of what is happening around them. When the mediation therapist understands the value of both types of seeing, he or she will be able to share the value of seeing clearly with his or her mediation therapy clients. Inasmuch as language and words have tremendous power, pictures—both internal and external—may be worth the proverbial thousand words in this intervention. Drawing what they see on a large easel in my office seems to help couples improve their pure seeing and visualization abilities, and the products are typically used as information in the creative problem-solving process.

Dream Images

The pictures that individual members of a couple generate in their nighttime dreams often indicate their inner concerns, contemporary and past. Dream interpretation, often assumed to be the province of individual psychotherapy or psychoanalysis, has great power in a couple forum such as mediation therapy. Long the road to discovery of one's interior wisdom, wishes, and intuition, dreams may be interpreted by mates in the context of mediation therapy in the same way visualizations are.

Deborah Luepnitz, in a recent talk, alluded to encouraging partners to interpret or guess at meanings and symbolism in one another's dreams.[11] These nighttime pictures are often very valuable in the mediation therapy context. Drawing pictures of dream sequences on the large easel is a fantastic medium for helping individuals translate dream images into understanding.

Body Signals

Words, images, dreams, pictures all convey knowledge to individuals and to partners, but only if they are attended to, only if they are respected as givers of knowledge. Many people respond favorably to learning how to recognize their internal cues and feelings. They enjoy learning to bring clues/cues to awareness as a first step in understanding the messages in their dreams, images, and body (kinesthetic) signals.

Questions such as the following may help people contact their body cues:

When you think about the difficulties in your relationship over the past X years, do you notice any feelings in your body?

Are the knots in your stomach fear, for certain? Could they be conflict, or tension, or even a sense of adventure?

When you visualize a future together, how do you feel?

Can you leave the past and the future visualizations out of awareness, for the most part, now, and be present with your awareness of the just now?

What does your body tell you about yourself just now? These questions are invaluable inspirations from neurolinguistic programming. The questions include specific requests to have the part of the person with the internal feeling communicate to the rational mind the message of the feeling. In Bandler and Grinder's words:

> One of the ways people really get into trouble is that they play psychiatrist with their own parts without being qualified. They interpret the messages they get from their own parts. So they begin to feel something and they name it "fear" when it may be some form of excitement, or some kind of aliveness or anything. By naming it and acting as if that is the case, they misinterpret communication externally.[12]

One mediation therapy client learned to listen to the numbness, the nothingness, not of a body part, but of his whole experience. As a soldier, he had seen a lot of conflict in Vietnam and talked about having blanked out his war experience upon return home. This dissociated sense of himself estranged him greatly from himself, his wife, and others. When asked by the mediation therapist if he could be in touch with the parts of himself that were aware and alive during those years, the veteran said that he could. Asked to speak to that part of himself, he said, crying, "I am so damned glad that you're alive." It was the beginning of his

regaining lost aspects of himself.

People in difficult situations—war or bad marriages that feel like war—do

tend to overlook, deny, and distort the traumatic experiences. Helping them

contact aspects of themselves in a limited way through the body is a part of

mediation therapy that is often excluded from traditional interventions for

assisting couples and families in crisis. Psychoanalysis, devised in Victorian times,

often behaves as if patients or clients have no bodies to check in with, only psyches

and the unconscious.

Emotional Sharing

The business of mediation therapy is to help people become aware of the many cues

readily available to them, including those within their bodies. Although mediation

therapy may appear to be predominantly a rational or cognitive intervention, with a great deal of structure and control by the mediation therapist, emotional

sharing, sensory discovery, and discharge of intense feelings occur frequently and

often at considerable depth. When one of the rational structures is being employed,

intense feelings of loneliness, abandonment, or rage may surface, and it is appropriate

to deal with these feelings then and there. For example, the rational impertinent

question "What bothers you most about your partner?" may be answered. "X works

seventy-five hours per week." Along with the expression of dissatisfaction, a surge of

intense emotions may accompany the rational response being worked on.

More often than not, emotional sharing and discharge occur with certain of the

rational structures. I believe one of the chief reasons for the evocation of strong

feelings in mediation therapy is that the rational structure bounds the feelings. It is

clear to people that they won't be overwhelmed or swept away by the intensity of

their emotion. They are allowed, even encouraged, to feel the emotions—rage,

sadness, disappointment—sharply and

deeply, and they sense that they will be returned to rational understanding.

Not only do our clients need to be aware of the emotions within themselves, they need to interpret them as accurately as I they can. Acquiring sensory information through eyes, ears, bodies, intuition, and inner wisdom is a necessary precursor to communication with any other person. Lack of inner awareness, of self-knowledge, can only lead to distorted and faulty communication. If a person isn't aware of him or herself, he or she can only speak about the other or the self from a place of incomplete awareness and self-knowledge, rather than from a positive place of self-knowledge.

Communication Skills

Paraphrasing

As previously touched on, paraphrasing is one is the most powerful tools of mediation therapy; it is a way of helping people become aware of what they know, think, and perceive. Paraphrasing may be viewed as taking the probable essence of what someone has said and repeating it calmly to the partner— without menacing gestures or intonation—all the while checking out with the communicator if what you've said was his or her intention. Metacommunication, or the implied message conveyed through tone and body language, is often included in the paraphrase.

Paraphrasing literally translates the person's intended message. In contrast, reframing, another therapeutic tool, attempts a *positive* translation of the message. At the beginning of the mediation therapy, it is a requirement for the mediation therapist to explain the process of paraphrasing, indicating that it involves guesswork on the part of the mediation therapist: "If the words fit, wear them and nod or say yes; if they don't, shake your head or say no." In mediation therapy two critical ways of helping couples begin to hear one another are:

1. paraphrasing

2. staying focused on individuals—that is, not allowing a
couple initially to jump into their repetitive patterns of communication.

Early on in mediation therapy, people will frequently mention an inability to communicate effectively. This is an ideal time to begin teaching them communication skills. The first part of teaching communication skills is always to attempt to assist the individuals to become aware of themselves, using both rational and sensory structures. Only when they have contacted some essential parts of themselves can individuals begin to think about learning communication skills. The object of knowing oneself within the partnership, at the time of the mediation therapy, is to be able to share one's realities with the other, to be known and understood.

Gender and Communication

In *Love Is Never Enough* Aaron Beck talks about

communication training. Never is he more compelling than when he speaks about the "different meanings of talk." Every couples therapist, every member of a heterosexual couple, cannot help but resonate to Beck's description that many women's attitudes are that "The marriage is working as long as we can talk about it," contrasted with many men's views that "The relationship is not working as long as we keep talking about it."[13]

What bridges does one build to breach this gap between these paradoxical meanings of talk? Bridging the differences between "subcultures" must start with making these differences apparent to the members of a partnership. It seems critical to me that men and women understand that talking means something like connectedness, reassurance, and viability to some women, while it may be a threat to some men, meaning that the relationship may not be viable. When he views her talking, and talking, he must learn to see that she is trying to connect, to be reassured; when she views his being silent, she must understand that he is content, there is nothing critical to discuss.

Beck states, "Women frequently want their partner to be a new, improved version of their best friend[14]." He says that men view their partners often as their best friends. He calls attention to men's propensity toward finding solutions, while women ofteh desire to be emphatically listened to and so feel hurt and slighted when presented with solutions. A tremendously important gender difference, cited by Beck, is in what men and women regard as important in what their mates tell them. The example Beck gives to illustrate this is a lawyer friend of his

> whose wife works in an art gallery, complains that she always wants to tell him the trivial details of who said what to whom while he would like to hear more about the kinds of paintings she is dealing with, her evaluation of them, and specific business details, such as purchasing strategies. He wants the facts and does not see the importance of his wife's conversations with her colleagues. To his wife, however; what happens between her and her associates at the gallery constitutes the fabric of her working life[15]."

If these differences between men and women make them like different subcultures, different nationalities, or even different races during different epochs, bridges between them would seem to be to understand those differences and pay respect to them, rather than attempts at conversion. Bridges might be created by joining with the other in his or her rituals— for example talking or not talking. Equality between subcultures is not sameness of the subcultures. Although some qualities may be voluntarily adopted by men or by women from each other, they are unlikely to be adopted through coercion. Certainly, when a man or a woman makes the gesture to communicate in a way that is specific to the other gender, that act may well have positive effects within the partnership.

Understanding and respecting gender differences, in general and in communication in particular, seems critical to good communication between members of different subcultures. Women need to respect men, to understand how they communicate differently. Likewise, men need to respect and not fear the differences in their partner's communication. These seem to be necessary first steps to effective communication between the sexes.

Listening

Another, sometimes invisible, step in really learning how to communicate is to perceive the immense power of listening to hear, to understand, to connect. Merely saying what one thinks and what one feels (so overvalued by novitiate therapy clients and sometimes by their psychotherapists) does not connect a person to any other person.

Genuine listening, with acknowledgment, is necessary before the spark of communication may take place. I make the following kinds of statements to a couple in the service of education about hearing, the very active, paradoxically receptive part of a communication:

"To listen is to have a quiet mind, to focus on what the
          other is saying and how he or she is feeling; not associating to your
own concerns."

"To hear is to understand what has been said, especially
          when you don't agree."

"One should not avoid listening when one anticipates that

the other is going to say something with which the listener disagrees." "If I know that circumstances will require my onging interaction with another person [ ] then I should continue to deal with them now even if I disapprove of their conduct."[16]

―

"And it is critical that we acknowledge what we have

heard."

Determination to keep a clean channel open to hear what is going on around one is a learned skill. People may be reminded that it may be over many years that they have been partially listening to, or listening very little to what is going on around them and that great efforts at concentration may be required in order to relearn the simple art of hearing.

Nonverbal Signals

As stated previously, in *Frogs into Princes* Bandler and Grinder talk about sensing, in addition to pure hearing: "If you clean up your sensory channels and attend to

sensory

experience, when you make a statement or ask a human being a question, they will always give you the answer non-verbally, whether or not they are able to consciously express what it is."[17] If an individual is open, he or she should be able to receive what has been said and to connect to the speaker; if the speaker has no understandable words, good "seeing" powers may often allow a listener to receive a powerful communication nonetheless. Listening to hear and sensing the answer when words don't come are the simple, yet complex tasks initially taught in the communication instruction sequence of mediation therapy.

Some questions may enable people to access sensory information:

"What strong feelings do you have at the present time?"

"What is the most compelling thing you have *heard* from
your partner in the last several weeks?"

"If you gave yourself permission to use your intuition,

what would you know?"

"If your relationship had little tension and conflict, how
would you feel?"

"What do you know from a place *deep within you* about
yourself, your partner, the relationship?"

"Do you feel responsible for the life, the health, the well
being of your partner?"

The mediation therapist, asking these questions to evoke her or his clients'
sensory observations, also uses her or his own senses to receive information that
mediation therapy clients are not yet ready or able to put into words.

Anger

More often than not, in addition to learning how to access sensory information,
couples need specific instruction in anger management and in assertiveness.
Uncovering their thoughts, feelings, and sensory observations gives them a wealth

of

information about themselves. Conveying what they've learned to their partners requires good communication skills, including the deft handling of anger and the positive assertion of thoughts and feelings.

Given that a couple has learned the modicum of communication skills taught in the first part of this chapter, the mediation therapist will often suggest that a couple read a short book by John Sanford, *Between People: Communicating One to One* or a longer one by Aaron Beck: *Love Is Never Enough.* Those people who don't feel they have time or predilection to read the suggested books and articles will not do so. However, people frequently express great recognition of themselves in the reading and great pleasure in recognition, however painful.

Asking each individual what, in particular, he or she resonated to in the reading seems to reveal some areas the individuals need to work on in themselves or in the relationship. Individuals frequently raise issues for discussion from the reading. If not, the mediation therapist might ask a couple what they think about Sanford's notion that hurt feelings, not expressed at the time, become larger.

The mediation therapist may point out her or his agreement with Sanford, that unexpressed emotions become larger and interfere with communication. Sanford says that rather than just *having* emotions, people frequently behave as if they had *become* their emotions. Mediation therapists try to teach clients to keep their feelings in proportion, remaining much larger than their emotions.

While giving instruction about communication to couples, some instruction about anger is helpful—for example, sharing the notion that there are many situations in which anger is a genuinely appropriate, normal response. In spite of what children may sometimes understand from parents, being angry does not, in any way make someone bad, undesirable, or unworthy. What one does with one's angry feelings, if socially unacceptable or hurtful to others (for example, hitting and harming one's siblings), is what parents often try to indicate is unacceptable. Unfortunately, children often perceive their angry feelings as bad rather than their subsequent behavior. Mediation therapists express the inevitability of having angry feelings and the necessity of expressing legitimately angry feelings in appropriate ways.

The mediation therapist suggest that people need to experiment. They need to discover what modes of expression satisfactorily discharge their emotion and enable them to move forward. Presenting a two-stage process of expressing anger— the toxic/ affective part first, then getting to an effective expression of the emotion— is productive. Does a person need a physical, visual or auditory outlet to express the toxic/affective part of anger? This stage of anger occurs when adrenalin is running high and a physical or a forceful release seems imminent. In private, some people need an auditory outlet such as screaming or making jungle noises; others need to write or draw their angry feelings, seeing them "out there" to gain perspective. Still others need physical, recreational, or a punching-bag outlet.

After the private outlet of the toxicity, when the adrenalin was running high, a verbal or written expression of anger is much easier and evolves into the stage of an effective expression of angry feelings. Role playing effective methods of expressing angry feelings provides an excellent learning experience.

During this time of instruction about anger, the deliberate physical, visual, or auditory expression of toxic/affective levels of anger is encouraged but clearly differentiated from the nondeliberate acting out of one's feelings by behaving in avoidant, hurt, and angry ways.

Assertiveness

Instruction in assertive communication may be blended with some of the structures in mediation therapy. For example, the mediation therapist may ask the couple one of the rational structures: "What are the aches, gripes, conflicts, and anxieties between you at this point?" The therapist may then add: "Think about the ways you now know to *assertively* communicate your message so that your partner may genuinely hear you."

Many of the rational structures, described in detail in chapter 4, are interesting, sometimes provocative questions that the couple answers individually and together. Since they are naturally engaged in mutual questioning already, interweaving principles of good communication is like jumping aboard a moving sidewalk.

Talk of assertiveness is interwoven with the discussion of good communication. Unfortunately, many people associate assertiveness with aggressiveness, which may mean to be actively hostile. One of the meanings of assertiveness is to express or state something positively—even though the expression may involve unpleasant, angry, disappointing messages. Assertive messages are received more kindly, by far, than aggressive

messages. Alternative modes of expression are the passive, do-nothing response, and

the passive/aggressive, wait-to-see or get-even response. For example, a prominent

person in your church or temple asks you, a woman, to bake cookies for a youth group

coming from out of town. The range of responses follows:

An assertive response: "I would like to be able to bake
cookies. Right now, while I'm working on this book and helping my
son get off to college, I am totally focusing on these things. I would be happy
to buy some cookies."

An aggressive response: "I don't bake cookies, for anyone,
church or temple, not anyone!"

A passive response: Bake the cookies at 2 A.M. while
writing and crying.

Passive/aggressive response: Bake the cookies. Later
spread the word widely that the person who asked you is an anti-
feminist throwback to a bygone era.

Not surprisingly, many people haven't an inkling about composing assertive responses, relying heavily on the other three alternatives to communicate with one another.

Education about assertiveness and communication, negotiation, disagreement, and decision making are vital components of mediation therapy. I tell couples that to be assertive is not to be hostile, but to be self-confident, clear with oneself and others, and respectful of others. Assertiveness is stating what one needs to say, positively, in a way the other is able to hear. Assertiveness is not an attempt to control, it is being firm, forceful, noncritical, affirming of oneself and the other, positive, and even tempered. In mediation therapy couples are taught to be assertive, to use all of their senses and taught a wide range of communication skills—as a part of assisting them in making sane, important decisions.

Notes

[1]

Bandler and Grinder, *Frogs into Princes,* 46.

[2] Ibid., 17.

[3] Erickson, *Wisdom and the Senses,* 26.

[4] Ibid., 25.

[5] Ibid., 79.

[6] Belenky et al., *Women's Ways of Knowing,* 129-130.

[7] Ibid., 133.

[8] Bandler and Grinder, 15.

[9] Ibid., 184.

[10] Ibid., 55.

[11] Deborah Luepnitz, "The Therapist and the Minotaur" lecture.

[12] Bandler and Grinder, 142.

[13] Beck, *Love Is Never Enough,* 83-84.

[14] Ibid., 84..

[15] Ibid., 84-85.

[16] Fisher and Brown, *Getting Together,* 5.

[17] Bandler and Grinder, 17

Conflict Negotiation Skills: The Cornerstone of Mediation Therapy

Conflict lies not in objective reality, but in people's heads. . . . The reality as each side sees it constitutes the problem in a negotiation and opens the way to a solution.

—Roger Fisher and William Ury, *Getting to Yes: Negotiating*

Agreement Without Giving In [1]

Seeing One's Own and the Other's Point of View

If the central problem in a negotiation is the way in which each partner sees

the conflict, then helping the partners see the other's point of view is the solution.

This is a central goal in mediation therapy—to help an individual see the other's

perceptions. Psychotherapy skills alone, without conflict-resolution skills, are not

enough to help couples learn to see and understand each other's viewpoints, nor are

they enough to assist couples in intense conflict to make

217

important once-in-a-lifetime decisions for their families.

The family therapist Yetta Bernard illustrates the importance of point of view in the following case.

"Now tell me . . . how *do you see* the problem in your relationship?" the psychotherapist asks the wife in the couple she is just beginning to meet with. The woman responds that her husband does not want to discuss issues about how the children from his first marriage don't listen to her. The psychotherapist paraphrases what the woman has said, asking her if she, the therapist, has heard the woman correctly.

When the woman nods affirmatively, the therapist turns to the husband, querying, "And, is how she puts it congruent with how you see the problem?"

"No!" responds the husband. It isn't that he doesn't want to discuss his children's behavior; but for him, it is a matter of timing. He would prefer not to discuss the matter every evening just as he is arriving home from work.[2] —

As Bernard's case shows so well, the problem in conflict is how people see the issues, not what the issues are or are not about. This couple both wanted to discuss his children's treatment of her; they differed in when to do so. Initially, she believed that he wasn't interested in discussing the children's treatment of her. After Bernard reframed the issue to be how each person separately saw the problem, the couple began to see the commonality in their interests.[3]

—

Because how individuals see the issues is critical for couples, many strategies in mediation therapy are perceptual/visual/seeing techniques, designed to assist individuals in finding and defining their own points of view. The techniques obviously must also help individuals see how their partner views a myriad of situations.

The mediation therapist needs to translate some of the

perceptual techniques into auditory or kinesthetic equivalents so that a large number of people who process information in ways that aren't visual may understand their partner's point of view. Regardless of the dominant sense through which people process information, "seeing" in mediation therapy is a process of uncovering, then discovering how one views an issue or a problem oneself.

After an initial self-discovery, seeing means assertive communication of one's viewpoint without accusation to the partner. Communication continues until the partner sees and thoroughly understands one's viewpoint, as the above couple finally understood that they each wanted very much to discuss an issue about the children, but that they were in disagreement about when to do so.

Basic Techniques of Conflict Resolution

Symmetry and Neutrality

Even before couples like the above are seen in the office for the first time,

the mediation therapist begins using basic techniques   of   conflict   negotiation

and   mediation. The development of a neutral stance (see chapter 2) is begun when

the mediation therapist requests that the caller's mate or significant other also

place a call (making a total of two phone calls) to the therapist to find out about the

intervention and to ask any questions. As previously stated, the therapist is not

contaminated as being the choice of the first caller.

This symmetrical balance and neutral stance are mediation techniques.

When equipoise is achieved before the couple even arrives in the office, their

mediation therapist is indicating that discussion and negotiation needs to be between

equal partners and that to facilitate discussion she or he needs to be neutral, receiving

symmetrical input from each of them.

The foundation for the resolution of conflicts in mediation therapy is equal,

balanced, information giving, with equal time

and attention devoted to each partner. Some clients in mediation therapy take longer than others to realize that their monopolizing time throws the entire process off-balance.

Speaking with both individuals prior to the session, the mediation therapist implicitly conveys to her or his clients that they will be empowered equally to participate fully and democratically in the process. Each will know that he or she is expected to be an active and equal participant in the process. This expectation of equality has often not been the case within the relationship. It will take many minor and major corrective actions within the sessions before a balance between the individuals even comes close to being achieved. The most obvious correction is the mediation therapist's stopping a loquacious person, over and over again, in order to achieve some symmetry in the volume of communication between individuals. The mediation therapist must risk the appearance of impoliteness to address the assymmetry. She or he must be firm: one of them is talking more than the other. She or he asks both of them to practice suspending their thoughts, to listen attentively, actively, and receptively to the other.

Symmetry in the volume of verbal communication is probably more important than symmetry in any other aspect of mediation therapy. When one person's excessive talking is felt as domination or control, the other mate is likely to be furious and inattentive. Excessive talking may also be intellectualization, having little to do with a person's true feelings, and it may consequently result in the partner's not paying attention. These locked-in patterns of unequal communication are interrupted by the mediation therapist's conviction that this kind of assymmetry in verbal production obviates mutuality, reciprocity, and real dialogue between intimate partners.

As a neutral professional, the mediation therapist must intrinsically understand that partners very often have oppositional positions and viewpoints, which may have truth for each individual. For a mediation therapist, looking for right or wrong positions, or better or worse positions, is fatal. Neutrality would be lost from the outset. The mediation therapist must be able to think in nuances, grays, individual truths, and trade-offs.

Neutrality is necessary in order to not get caught in a couple's polarizations, in their black and white thinking. The mediation therapist needs to help couples understand that she or he is not with or for individuals, but for a good, workable solution for both people and for their family. Stating each individual's goal at the outset of the process serves the function of establishing symmetry and equality and helps the mediation therapist preserve a neutral stance.

Developing Improved Communication

"I" Statements. The mediation therapist carefully structures the beginning phase of the process to avoid starting on the wrong foot. As previously mentioned, it is not desirable to begin the process with what is wrong with one person or the relationship. It is desirable to begin with nonaccusatory "I" statements, which are an integral part of this conflict negotiation approach: what each individual, for her or himself, wants to accomplish in this process. The person who has said, "You never take vacations with me!" might translate the accusation into "Will you come to the Seychelles with me this summer?" From the inception of the process, the mediation therapist explicitly conveys a basic principle of mediation therapy—not to blame, not to accuse. However, accusations do get made. That is why turning accusations into requests is necessary.

We ask a great deal of mediation therapy clients. We ask that they become aware of their goals, their theories, their asymmetrical communications, and we ask the individuals to reach into a probable morass of intense feelings of rage, disappointment, sadness, and revenge—to articulate what they, as individuals, want to accomplish in the present. We ask them to step back into the rational parts of themselves, for the time being, to be an advocate for what they now need. We begin with hope, with what individuals want for themselves, not with their problems.

Paraphrasing. The mediation therapist is advised to frequently check out whether a second partner has heard what the first individual is saying. From the beginning, each partner is asked for his or her understanding of the other's goal for this intervention. When the goal is repeated, does the first partner agree with how the second one has restated his or her goal for the intervention?

Initially, funneling information through the mediation therapist has the advantage, with a couple in intense conflict, of allowing each individual to hear the other's viewpoint without the anger, negative body language, and repetitious negative meanings, which over time have come to be associated with the words. Many couples need the funneling of information through a therapist in the initial stages. Funneling of information means not allowing intensely angry individuals to talk directly to one another, initially. The mediation therapist functions as a fulcrum channeling the chaotic energy of the couple into constructive energy to help them move forward.

If individuals cannot talk without fighting, basic instruction is given in communication—in listening, hearing, acknowledging — and in assertiveness, the positive statement of a message. Most couples, not long after the instruction, can safely talk with each other without the funneling of information through the mediation therapist. Some couples speak directly to one another, clearly hearing one another from the inception of the process. Many couples fall somewhere in between, sometimes hearing one another, sometimes not. When the direct engagement of the couple in communication is counterproductive, the mediation therapist may ask them to wait a while, to learn some basic principles before attempting to communicate directly with one another. She or he indicates that she or he will paraphrase for them, checking out her correctness, until direct communication becomes possible.

For example, through the mediation therapist's use of the paraphrase, each member of one couple heard something new from the other that neither had heard in thirty years of marriage. The gentleman, in his fifties, was the only child of elderly parents. He had spent much time in reverie as a child and had developed an active imagination. No one in his childhood and adolescence had ever explicitly asked him to share his ideas or thoughts, let alone feelings. He was surprised to hear, through the paraphrase, that his wife had repeatedly been asking him to share his imaginations, thoughts, and feelings with her. He said to her: "I honestly didn't have a clue that you want to hear my thoughts."

She said to him, after hearing the therapist's paraphrase, "You know, in thirty years of marriage, I never understood that you feel intimidated by the amount that I talk. You've never said that before. You also never have said that you feel so inadequate verbally in comparison with me, nor have you ever said that you feel frightened nearly every time we talk. I am amazed."

Paraphrasing often reveals basic, important misunderstandings and miscommunications.

When the mediation therapist paraphrases, she says what she believes reflects the fundamental core of truth in what a person has said, checking out after she paraphrases if the meaning she conveyed was correct. The person who has spoken and has been paraphrased then indicates whether the paraphrase indicated his meaning or how he would modify the paraphrase to represent his own exact meaning.

Often enough, a spouse will reply, in response to a paraphrase, "Is that really what you have been trying to say all these years?" or, "I never knew you felt that way!" Paraphrasing is different from reframing, which gives a positive connotation to a statement in an effort to help people to hear. Paraphrasing adheres to the meaning exactly and attempts to refine the statement so that it becomes more clear to the listener.

To distinguish reframing from paraphrasing, the remark "You are such a slob," reframed might be "I love you in so many ways. I would feel much better about you if you tried to be neater"—a positive reframing. The same remark, paraphrased more literally by the mediation therapist, might be "Jon, Alice is saying that she feels you are not as neat as you might be."

Toward the outset of the intervention the mediation therapist explains that blaming and accusation are literally outlawed in this intervention. When they occurs she asks that the individuals turn those accusations or blaming into requests. When one partner says, "You never give my mother a call!" he is asked to turn that accusation into a request. He may say, "Could you please give my mother a call sometime this week?"

What so often blocks comprehension between mates? This most likely comes from a person feeling defensive, blamed, or accused by the other's statements, combined with a feeling of powerlessness to do anything about a situation the partner is describing. Why hear, if there is nothing one can do about the situation? Over time, people may make a habit of being inattentive to one another. Often people who have heard an abundance of negative statements in the past automatically hear statements as having negative tones in the present. People constantly criticized in the past tend to hear criticism in the present. Some people fear genuine intimacy with one another so that not hearing what could connect them to the other accomplishes a lack of intimacy. Hearing one another with empathy and understanding may be unconsciously feared, as, not only do hearing and understanding potentially move the partners toward intimacy, they also move them toward losses of other things important to the individual: control, identity, egoboundaries, privacy, space.

Finally, the need to control the other's behavior, in lieu of self- control, or the attempt to clone one's own exquisite selfcontrol onto the other, may interfere with people hearing their partners as distinct individuals. It is small wonder that paraphrasing is so frequently necessary to help related people hear what they are saying to one another.

The initial use of paraphrasing by mediation therapists may be experienced by those therapists as audacious, as taking over for or speaking for their clients, possibly disempowering them. Experience proves the contrary. In mediation therapy a couple and their college-age daughter were discussing the parameters of their obligations, including financial responsibilities, with one another. Their conversation required extensive paraphrasing, to the point of literal exhaustion of the mediation therapist.

The immediate reaction of the mediation therapist, after the session, was to question: "What have I done? Have I spoken for all of them? Have I said what they meant?" Yet, each of the three of them had shaken hands with the mediation therapist as they left the office, expressing gratitude at having been able to understand one another for the first time. Paraphrasing can be like sign language, the tool that bridges between two modes of understanding. It may well prove to be the single most powerful tool in mediation

therapy. It defuses anger, thereby allowing a couple to hear one another, and also

proscribes old, repetitive, destructive patterns of communication, which impede

the resolution of the conflict. The visible relief that occurs when a person perceives

that she or he has been interpreted in a way her or his partner can hear is visual

demonstration of the power of the paraphrase.

Instruction in Disagreement

Paraphrasing frequently reveals early in the process that the individuals are not in

accord in their beliefs. This discordance frequently causes discomfort for the

partners. For this reason, education about disagreement begins almost

immediately in mediation therapy. The mediation therapist will establish what the

individuals believe to be true about disagreement in couples: Is any disagreement

between partners acceptable or not? If it is not acceptable to either partner, an educational process about disagreement begins. I often make the following points:

We are not striving for consensus here, nor do we expect
it.

We are striving for each of you to understand the other,
his or her viewpoints and attitudes.

From understanding each other, I hope to help you learn
to negotiate to some mutually acceptable solutions.

For one of you to get your needs met, the other absolutely
does not have to sacrifice his or her needs.

You both win, in terms of getting your needs met and
being understood.

When a couple is able to constructively state their disagreement, the mediation

therapist shows them that they now have the option of learning to negotiate those

differences. Or they may put the disagreement on the record, opting simply to register

it or put a disagreement on the back burner for later

negotiation. Where putting aside of disagreement methods are used, the mediation therapist may point out that the couple has together reached an agreement about what to do: the disagreement will not be immediately negotiated. This instruction in disagreement is one of five instructional methods used in mediation therapy. Others on assertiveness, communication, negotiation, and decision making are detailed in other chapters.

The actual subject being discussed when instruction in disagreement seems appropriate may be almost any subject: answering the rational inquiries; the individuals' looking at themselves; dealing with intense feelings that have accumulated over a long period of time. These instructional techniques are used throughout the mediation therapy process.

Radical Conflict Resolution Techniques

Radical conflict resolution techniques are used when

emotions run high.

1. The mediation therapist may insist on only one person
   speaking at a time.

2. She or he may suggest taking a quarter-hour break for
   coffee or until the next session, saying, "The heat in the office is too
high, let's break until X time."

3. She or he may say, "You're right on your toes, thinking
   fast, but let's take some time out to spell out some ground rules for
our discussions."

4. Sometimes the mediation therapist might wisely rise,
   walk around the room, sit between the partners or may even leave
the office until the "temperature" decreases.

The process of mediation therapy obviously will not require these basic
conflict negotiation techniques or instructions at all times. Throughout the entire
process, outbursts of conflict will occur that necessitate the use of these techniques.

Case Study in Negotiation:

Taking a look at the negotiation process—from the vantage point of a specific couple and their mediation therapist, who are in the process of mediating some important conflicts—will serve to bring alive the above discussion of the basic conflict negotiation techniques in mediation therapy.

At the point when we enter their process, Peter Andrews is making it clear that he has indeed understood that the mediation therapy is a neutral process. He is saying that he is aware that his wife also spoke on the telephone to the mediation therapist prior to the first appointment, sharing her own perception of their situation. He continues by saying that his goal for the mediation therapy is to understand whether there is any hope of salvaging their marriage. He believes that Sonja, his wife of one year from whom he has been separated for one month, has heard his goal and he understands that she is terribly threatened by it.

Likewise, he has heard that her goal is a different one: she wants very much to be married, to resume living together immediately, a goal that feels threatening to Peter's autonomous sense of himself. The mediation therapist has said repetitively that it is fine for couples to have different goals. It is of primary importance to understand the other person's goal and how the other is looking at a variety of issues.

Peter Andrews outwardly seems perplexed and irritated that his wife is declaring so boldly that she wants to be married to him; inwardly he is pleased to be wanted. He appeared grateful for the opportunity to tell his wife that the reasons he left her were irrational and unfounded jealousy and her powerful attempts to control him; from what kind of soup he should order in the Japanese restaurant, to forceful attempts on Sonja Andrews's part to prevent him from going out socially with his male friends.

The mediation therapist asked Sonja to repeat why her

husband left, and what feelings he had demonstrated upon leaving. Her initial

understanding wasn't close to her husband's reasoning, but became closer each

time she stated his motivation. Peter finally looked certain that his wife understood

why he left and how angry he was about her attempts to control him, as well as how

provoked he became by her unfounded jealousy. He learned, for the first time, that she

had many times before been left by boyfriends who had become infuriated by her self-

avowed manipulative jealousy.

Peter heard, and wanted to believe, that his wife was genuinely interested in

working hard to discontinue her jealous responses. The biggest surprise for Peter,

however, was in learning that Sonja considered many of her controlling actions to be

the kinds of caring directives one gives to the loved ones in one's family and in the

culture in which she grew up: if you care about someone, you advise them of the best

soup on the menu. To Peter, if you care about someone, you refrain from any

suggestion that would even appear to interfere with a person's individual rights.

Peter's head was spinning after the initial round of discussion. He felt Sonja understood his goal for mediation therapy and he knew that he understood hers. He was clear that she finally understood why he left, and that she understood he was furious. He was surprised that she acknowledged responsibility for what was primarily angering him, her unfounded jealousy. And he was surprised that she claimed she wanted to change. The confusing part to him was that he and Sonja were not experiencing the "controlling" behaviors in the same way: Sonja felt she was expressing caring in a way her cultural background prescribes when telling him, for example, which soup to order. He felt this behavior as powerful attempts to control him and felt that his autonomy was being threatened.

The mediation therapist has bent over backwards to make disagreements in perception acceptable. Peter Andrews decides to go along with this formulation about the controlling

240

behaviors, even though he is feeling fairly hopeless about Sonja's actions changing enough for him to feel comfortable with her. Nothing has changed to this point for Peter, but he feels that he and Sonja better understand each other's behavior in the marriage and both understand why they are living separately.

At a similar point, Sonja Andrews is relieved to acknowledge her irrational jealousy, to acknowledge her desire to work on her behavior and to save the marriage. Sonja is very frightened; the man she has chosen "for life" is saying that he is not at all sure he wants the marriage. She is sure that her goal is to stay married; down deep she is furious that he could even question being married to her. This is just one more time in her life when her hard-working attempts to control another person are simply not working. She feels impotent and scared. She feels as though the sky is falling down upon her when her husband talks about her jealousy.

This manipulative pattern of jealousy unquestionably exists, has manifested itself in many previous relationships and is finally acknowledged by Sonja. At first, she feels cornered, then relieved. However, the controlling behaviors that her husband talks about are the same behaviors her mother and grandmother exhibited to show their husbands their caring. And, if she weren't feeling so guilty about her jealousy, she would have expressed how frustrating her husband's excessive need for space and privacy were for her. (This she eloquently expressed later on.)

Sonja Andrews believes that her viewpoint is the right way to look at the matter, and believes that her whole cultural group perceives directives as construing caring. She is now hearing from the mediation therapist that there is no right way or wrong way of viewing issues, only his way and her way, which need to be understood by the other. Sonja hears the mediation therapist saying that every couple disagrees, and hears her extolling the value of disagreement, which may be negotiated to solutions that Sonja and her husband both can contribute to and both may accept.

It sounds better to Sonja to simply have the same point of view about everything: maybe her parents had been right after all about the preference for, even necessity of, marriage within the same cultural group. Gradually, over time, Sonja comprehends that her husband, given his professional orientation, his own ethnic and cultural background, and so forth, simply does see things differently than she does. She finally, legitimately, understands how he might have come to those different viewpoints, and accepts that she might have to indicate her caring in a more direct way, along with clearly stating a "mere suggestion" regarding the best soup in the house.

Parenthetically, Peter also, over time, honestly begins to understand that his wife's behaviors, which he experiences as controlling, are positively connoted behaviors in the cultural milieu in which his wife grew up. When she slips and says, "Have the miso soup," he understands she is being caring and not controlling.

After seeing and accepting the other's viewpoint, as the Andrews did, the need arises for the development of a mutually acceptable solution, an "our viewpoint." To get from point A, seeing the other's viewpoint, to point Z, a mutually acceptable solution, instruction in communication and negotiation were required.

Acknowledgment,   fundamental   principle
                   a   in
communication, is modeled by the mediation therapist and explicitly explained to each couple. After instruction, when Sonja says "Have the miso soup!" Peter acknowledges that he hears her suggestion, is grateful for her expertise in Japanese cuisine and for her caring that he order something he will like. Sonja, knowing that her intentions have been heard and understood through her husband's acknowledgment, then demonstrated a repeated ability to attend to her husband's thoughts and positions.

Along with paraphrasing, teaching individuals

communication skills is one of the most important tools in mediation therapy. These

communication skills may include:

slowing down and acknowledging what the other is
saying

becoming aware of behaviors that are habitual

practicing discipline, sacrificing personal responses such
as interruption

attending and being present with the other.

Very important for couples to understand is that being receptive to hearing

one another is, indeed, an active, powerful response. Each individual is requested to

practice timing his or her responses to when the other would most likely be able to

hear them—that is, to hold off communication until fertile ground is available on

which to plant the seeds.

Teaching Negotiation Skills

Some modicum of listening and communication skills is critical for people to even begin using a verbal intervention to make a decision about the future of their relationship or other important matter. At a point at which couples can hear one another, can acknowledge what they've heard, and can communicate their thoughts and feelings back and forth without accusation, the mediation therapist begins to teach negotiation skills. Many of these skills will already have been modeled by the mediation therapist in an attempt to manage the couple's conflicts. The mediation therapist prefaces the formal instruction in negotiation by acknowledging that the couple, in all likelihood, already knows and employs some of these same techniques in other areas of their lives.

Preliminary to the negotiation, I begin conflict negotiation instruction by sharing with the couple my self-knowledge equation:

Self-Knowledge Equation

O	=	*optimal* solution for me *not*
N	=	*acceptable* solutions for me
/	=	development of *acceptable*
	=	solutions
A		
A		

To negotiate, each person needs to be in touch with him or herself, knowing which solution would be optimal for him or her. He or she needs to know, as well, the solutions he or she could not live with. Too often, people negotiate only with optimals, not understanding that there might be acceptable solutions. Going head to head with optimal solutions is to say "This has got to go my way." Under the line, in the equation, on the bottom-line position, each person will develop a series of acceptable solutions. Armed with this self-knowledge, and not before, an individual can begin to make proposals to the other in an effort to reach mutual solutions. He can accept her proposal, or make counterproposals, then add modifications, ad infinitum, until a mutually acceptable solution or several acceptables are found. To offer an image of this process: a new raindrop is formed that combines several raindrops from the now-melting icicles of the impasse.

Often brainstorming—exploring many and diverse, even ridiculous-sounding options—will lead to a solution with which both individuals can live. As stated by Ira Gorman, "the most important part of the process is for the brainstormer to let down his [or her] censor and put down everything that comes to mind. Any good list of brainstormed ideas will contain many wild ones."[4] Gorman illustrates the brainstorming process used with a single individual attempting to determine his future direction:

Mr. Black's Options or Ideas

1. Divorce

2. Live alone for trial separation 3. Move

in with an old friend

4. Six-month marriage counseling contract 5. Separate

bedrooms

6. Strict contract with rules to live at home

7. Have employer transfer [him] to another city for three

months

8. Work in Europe for a year and bring family 9. Individual

therapy for both partners

10. Family therapy with a well-known family therapist 11. Make clear

commitment to act differently 12. Join commune

13. Suicide

This man ranked his considerations for making his decisions as follows:

Considerations	Importance in Numbers
Children's welfare	5
Financial security	2
End the fighting	4
Freedom to pursue interests	3

After weighting his considerations, Mr. Black correlates his options with these

important considerations. This assigning of numerical weights to the considerations is

originally seen in the work of Robin Dawes in *Rational Choices in an Uncertain World.*

[5]

The mediation therapist may or may not want to contribute ideas and options to the

brainstorming process. When introducing brainstorming, Fisher and Ury's *Getting*

to Yes: Negotiating Agreement Without Giving In is an excellent reference for

couples. The mediation therapist may choose to share with clients sections from

books and articles about brainstorming and the negotiation process in general.

Since emotions are often very high at this point, some people readily use intellectual

information to defuse intensity, to gain distance through information. For other

people, the last thing they want to do at this juncture is to read any books, let alone

one on conflict, in which they are already amply immersed. Those who do take the recommendation to incorporate reading into their process generally report highly favorably about its efficacy for them.

As I have stated repeatedly, it is important for couples to understand that one person doesn't have to be wrong for the other person to be right; often enough, people have oppositional positions, both with veracity. One person doesn't need to lose, or to be deprived, for the other to have his or her needs met. These are essential attitudes for individuals to have for negotiations to be successful. Couples need to understand at the outset that mediation therapy can mostly be a process of mutual gain. In coming to the process, they have already reached a fundamental decision together: they have agreed to end a state of limbo, agreed to make a decision about the future direction of their relationship. Additionally, the couple needs to see the conflict that brought them to this point as an opportunity to reach a decision, to move forward constructively with their lives, together or apart, at home or away.

I request a change in perspective of the person who is feeling that he or she is "giving in" by giving up an original position: "Can you see this change as *not giving up*, but as creating something new, a new solution together? Can you see this finding of a mutual solution as generating not just one concrete solution, but as generating *a process* that will be concrete stepping stones to the resolution of many future conflicts?

The diagram shown in figure 6—1, which hangs in my office, was worked out with a class in conflict resolution. It illustrates an important distinction between conflicts and problems. As is evident in this diagram, understanding that the conflicts are not the problem helps those in conflict address the problem directly without becoming mired in their conflicting positions.

Figure 6.1 Differentiating the Problem from the Conflict

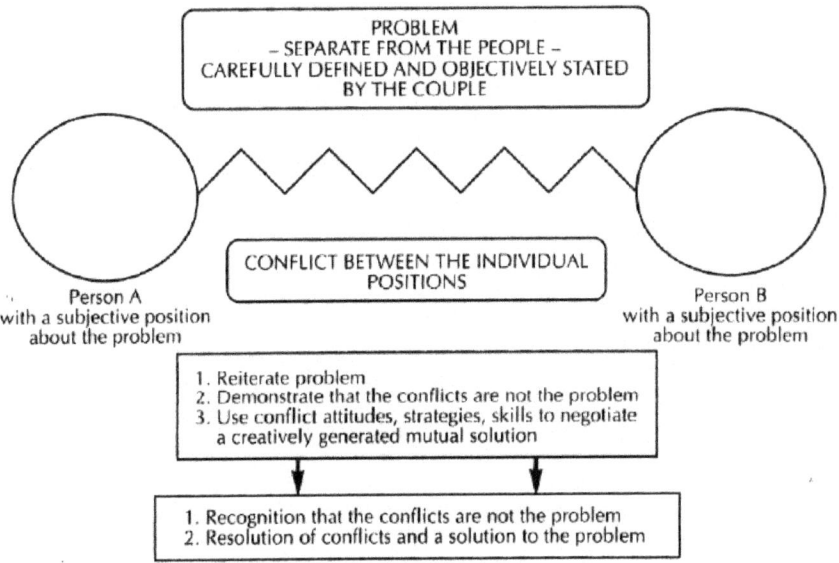

To illustrate the negotiation process further, a second couple beginning

mediation therapy, Chris and Bill, were polarized around strong positions; she

wanted to be married soon, he definitely did not want to get married soon. Ferreting

out their underlying interests revealed that neither wanted to marry before they

were both really sure of their decision. Through the mediation therapy process

they decided to live together for one year, which she had initially opposed as implying a lack of commitment. She accepted the living together plan, with the proviso that at the one-year point they would decide whether to become engaged. This plan staged a commitment over time. The negotiation outcome addressed their joint interest in feeling a larger degree of certainty in making their marriage commitment.

Separation and divorce are frequently seen as defeat. Having a family member live in an institutional residence is also frequently seen as defeat. Some other ways of looking at these situations are as opportunities for independent growth; for appropriate socialization with peers of one's age; or as a way of understanding that there are needs and responsibilities that could not be met in the marriage or at home.

The mediation therapist helps the couple to see conflict and their options constructively. She or he teaches the couple conflict resolution techniques and attitudes, directly and indirectly, by using them. Using the concepts of Fisher and Ury, the mediation therapist looks beneath the couple's stated positions, to their interests, helping them look for opportunities for mutual gain.

Being fair and reasonable with each other and themselves is an option the mediation therapist keeps in full view, especially when a couple seems to be competing for control or for the "goods" in their relationship. Phrases such as "one fair solution might be" put ownership of an idea into the fairness camp, not into either one of the individual's camps.[6] People are taught that they can get back to the other, that they don't have to make decisions exactly at the time that proposals are made. Decisions and conflicts can be shelved or put on the back burner.

To use another example, during the initial stages of an initial interview, while a couple was sharing their essential lists, the wife suddenly brought up an affair her husband had had fifteen years ago. I asked if such a critical, very important issue could be postponed until after the rational discussion of their needs was finished. If the wife had felt it was paramount to discuss the issue immediately, then her need would have been met. In this situation the wife was able to say she could postpone the discussion of the affair, and later seemed to bring a component of rationality into the discussion.

"Backing right out of that one for the moment, let's take up the matter of X," is a technique the mediation therapist may use to interrupt destructive communication. Couples in mediation therapy are often in high conflict. When one partner brings something up, the issue need not, as illustrated above, be discussed at that very moment.

On the other hand, Fisher and Ury's ventilation suggestion, encouraging an individual or an intensely angry person to continue until he or she is done, is the opposite strategy and is also frequently useful.[7] With this technique, people are encouraged to picture themselves on the same side of the table together, problem solving, with the problem on the opposite side of the table. As mentioned previously in the section on radical conflict resolution techniques, if badgering or antagonism gets too high, the mediation therapist may want to call for a short break, end the session, or stand up and leave the room, saying that when the heat decreases in the room it will be appropriate to continue.

Very occasionally, people posture to strike one another, or actually get up to do so. The mediation therapist, if brave, can stand between the couple, explaining that physical violence is out of the question. He or she can state that if it seems that it might arise again, the session will have to be discontinued. These radical conflict management techniques need rarely be used.

To a couple at loggerheads, the mediation therapist often explains that when we are in crisis we all typically think more narrowly and rigidly than usual. At this juncture of intense crisis the use of humorous brainstorming often helps loosen the rigidity in the thinking of partners: "What are your ideas, even very ridiculous ones, for breaking the logjam, or getting your thinking out of such tight boxes?"

All of the conflict approaches that combine into the mediation therapy conflict segment—Fisher and Ury's, Fisher and Brown's, Bernard's, Miller Wiseman's—seem to have some basic principles in common:

1. Each process gives people a chance to save face, preserving their individual dignity.

2. Each process helps people to identify their problems and to separate those problems from themselves as respected individuals.

3. Each process encourages brainstorming or the development of creative options.

4. In order to make decisions, each process requires some development and clarification of information.

5. Each approach also asks people to be specific: If she claims her partner is demented, she is asked to be

specific about how her partner exactly manifests being demented.

6. Each conflict approach demands that individuals find
their own position or viewpoint and acknowledge the other's point
of view.

7. Each approach uses some version of the paraphrase in
an effort to help supposed antagonists better hear one another.

In some manner all the approaches use the following techniques:

"I" statements

active, receptive listening

explicit/specific statements (be specific!)

acknowledgment of all feelings as legitimate double-

checking what was said
outlawing the blaming of others.

Yet the approaches also have distinct differences. One distinction between Yetta Bernard's and my own approach from Fisher and Ury's principled negotiation is that in Bernard's and my approaches, the differences between couples are often emphasized, while Fisher and Ury emphasize shared interests and look for commonalities. The question asked in mediation therapy, originally Bernard's question, "Are the differences between you a threat to your relationship?" seems an unlikely question for principled negotiators to ask. But, in mediation therapy, an assessment of differences between people, as well as their similarities, needs to take place before looking for joint interests.

Each of the conflict negotiation approaches imply commitment, but each has a different bottom line of commitment. For Yetta Bernard's approach the couples must have a bottom-line commitment to one another; for my approach the couples must have a commitment to the process of decision making; for Fisher and Ury's the couple must have a commitment to finding a solution for mutual gain.

Mediation therapy is different from principled negotiation in that it looks for differences between members of a couple, as well as commonalities. Mediation therapy has therapeutic aspects; it looks at resistances to resolving conflicts, at what people have invested in not resolving conflict, by virtue of unconscious needs, identity requirements, pride, or selfdefinition. The analysis of resistances, especially on an unconscious level, is not a part of principled negotiation.

Bernard's Contributions

Yetta Bernard's unique contributions to the mediation therapy conflict management approach have been the concepts of:

bottom-line and non-negotiable positions inalienable

rights

ground rules

role responsibilities

aches, gripes, conflicts, and anxieties

In addition, her suggestion to parents that they each have the power when they are dealing alone with their children helps parents act powerfully, alone, on their own authority, while overall policy making done together is the place where parents need to learn to pool their power and decision making as a united front.

Bernard's question, "Are the differences between you a threat to your relationship?" is a powerful question, which, as stated earlier, has frequent applicability in mediation therapy. It separates out the potentially relationship-destroying differences from real, but not lethal, differences. In addition, Bernard's technique of giving a partner an appointment within twenty-four hours to address a question that the second partner is not prepared to address is an approach needed for all couples, especially those in severe conflict. Bernard illustrates a technique of having a couple set up a time to discuss one person's burning issue when the other person doesn't have time to discuss it on the spot. For example, the couple mentioned early in this section learned to set up times to discuss her burning issues regarding the children other than when her husband arrived home in the evening.

Bernard's question: "Just *how far* apart do you think you are?" helps couples realistically assess the degree of difference between them.[8]

Principled Negotiation's Contributions

All of Fisher's and Ury's principled negotiation techniques and Fisher and Brown's many techniques are helpful for mediation therapists and their clients. The mediation therapist and sometimes her or his clients can benefit by reading *Getting to Yes: Negotiating Agreement Without Giving In*. The range of techniques and attitudes in principled negotiation is too broad to delineate here, but

this range includes:

active listening

acknowledging what is said positive

framing and reframing respect for the

other

finding joint interests for mutual gain generating

multiple options
brainstorming

hearing a position as one option personally

supporting the other person

One very important principle in principled negotiation, also central to mediation

therapy, is that completely understanding another's point of view is not the same as

agreeing with that viewpoint. Far too many people seem to believe that if they acknowledge that they've understood another, agreement with the other's person's position has been signaled. Not so. One can say: "I understand what you're saying, I agree with this part, but I take a different view on Y."

Fisher and Brown's book *Getting Together: Building a Relationship Which Gets to Yes* has, at minimum, two important principles for mediation therapy clients. The first principle is to do what is good for oneself and the relationship, without the expectation of return—that is, without expecting reciprocal behavior. For example, one partner might say, "I want to take us both to the museum for the exhibition," without expecting the other partner to reciprocate in any way at any other time.

The other principle useful for mediation therapy clients is to understand that the best way to be understood by the partner is to give up trying to be understood and to attempt to understand the partner.[9] Instead of saying "But, you're not understanding me, I mean ..." say "Please tell me what you mean exactly by . .."

Miller Wiseman's Contributions

Some of my unique contributions to my own conflict management integrated approach are:

the essential lists, which help individuals step back from
the morass of fighting, where they feel deprived and depleted, to identify what they want and need in any good, long-term relationship, what they will not tolerate, as well as what problems and strengths they bring to any good long-term relationship

asking individuals to convert accusations, criticisms, and
blaming into requests

identifying the realistic scope of a problem, large or small,
as a way to accurately define problems and solutions

using imagery, metaphors, and drawing pictures asking couples how their

own families—and the cultural

ethnic groups they grew up in—handled conflict, divorce, separation, anger, sadness, and disagreement

the self-knowledge equation.

With regard to questions about individual's cultural influences, individuals frequently respond, "I didn't exactly grow up in family of problem solvers. Come to think of it, neither did my parents or my grandparents." People at this stage may become sympathetic toward themselves regarding their feelings of not knowing the first thing about handling differences in opinion, belief, or values. Reviewing their familial, cultural models or context for the resolution of conflict may be helpful if they have good models or if they have had poor or no models for conflict resolution in their families. When they're asked to remember the first time they experienced another person satisfactorily resolving conflict, they often cite contemporaries, colleagues, or friends, in the recent past or present. For example, one mediation therapy client related that the first time she remembered seeing a conflict negotiated well was when she accompanied a colleague

to a store, where the colleague was intent upon exchanging a dress. The colleague

knew there was a no-return/no-exchange policy in this exclusive shop. After the

colleague found a more expensive dress that she liked, the colleague convinced the

store manager of the mutual gain they would experience in his making a larger sale

and in her getting the dress she wanted. This was the mediation therapy client's first

memory of an effective resolution to a conflictual experience.

Some people who haven't seen positive conflict resolution in their families remember

parents of friends who impressively negotiated their differences. Important to our

process is that people realize that just because they haven't grown up in families

of problem solvers doesn't mean they haven't had surrogate conflict negotiation

mentors or models in their environments. It is important to be able to say, "I want to

resolve conflicts as effectively, smoothly, or graciously as my friend

Andrea does. I've seen what I want to be able to do."

If people know and admire couples who effectively resolve their conflicts, or if they watch "The Cosby Show," for example, where negotiation is done regularly, these models will reinforce a couple's notions that effective conflict negotiation for them might well be possible. It is important to be able to visualize effective conflict resolution.

Resisting Conflict Resolution

Is this instruction in conflict negotiation, plus the instruction people get in their daily lives, enough to start couples negotiating effectively? For some couples it may be enough. For others, tapping into their resistances to resolving conflicts will be necessary. There must be myriad reasons why people resist resolving conflicts. Asking the bold question, "What is positive about keeping these conflicts going?" often nets an answer like Erik, a mediation therapy client, gave: "For me, the positive is that I get a sense of independence and space of my own. I think Ellen would manipulate me out of my space and independence if we were together on things and not in conflict all of the time."

Ellen also described the positives in being in conflict with Erik all the time: "I don't want to lose my own personal identity like I did in my first marriage. We were all 'wavy and mergy' but not as positively as Ward and June Cleaver. I'd rather be in conflict all the time than be the perfect couple with no individual identity."

The mediation therapist may comment compassionately and genuinely on the stake each member of the couple has in their conflict, perhaps by making a paradoxical statement such as, "From a personal standpoint, Ellen, it sounds as if you want and need very much to be your own person. From this viewpoint, you don't dare resolve these conflicts with Erik." To Erik, the mediation therapist could comment paradoxically: "It sounds like if you're going to continue to reassure your independence and have your own space, these conflicts are vital to you."

If the couple comes to understand the mutually exclusive nature of their thinking—they say they want to resolve conflicts on the one hand, but they have large stakes in not resolving conflicts, on the other hand—they may be ready to explore how to go about protecting individual needs, while achieving interdependence. The necessity of their ongoing repetitive conflicts may be lessened by exposing some of the underlying needs these conflicts serve.

Seeing how the conflict serves a function is an initial step. Actually having the couple close their eyes to see, hear, and feel what their internal and external environment might be like without excessive conflict is a next possible step. It is peaceful, empty, harmonious, boring, energizing? In other words, what do they imagine the ability to resolve conflicts will bring them? If resolving conflicts brings negative results, then their resistance to learning conflict resolution is at least partially understood by them. Why settle conflicts if some great loss will most likely follow?

Finally, the couple may be asked to think about how often they use avoidance, individually and together, as a method, or the primary method, for attempting to deal with conflict. The couple is asked to consider how effective avoiding conflict has been: does the avoidance method work well? Addressing a couple's resistances and avoidances to dealing with conflict— bringing out what they derive from having the conflicts and what is derived from avoiding them—is often essential to instruction in conflict resolution in mediation therapy.

The Andrews Revisited

To close the discussion of the conflict negotiation approach in mediation therapy, we will return to Peter and Sonja Andrews. When we last saw them, they had each achieved an understanding of how the other saw the problems. Sonja Andrews could

understand that her caring directives were actually perceived negatively by her

husband—as attempts to control him and limit his freedom. She already knew, too

well, that her jealousy and impulsive accusations were her own individual

problems, which she began to address by contemplating and beginning

individual psychotherapy.

Peter Andrews understood that his wife was bothered by her own impulsive,

jealous accusations, and that the caring directives, which he experienced as orders,

were behaviors his wife had learned in her family of origin as intended expressions of

caring. Nonetheless, as we look in on them, again, Peter still experiences those

behaviors as intensely controlling, no matter how they were intended in her family.

Peter and Sonja were able to use instruction and reading about relationships,

communication, and negotiation to talk about their relationship. They spent time

in their sessions

intensely communicating. They began to speak from   "I"

positions, moving away from their previously high levels of blaming and accusations. The mediation therapist firmly reinforced in a positive way when they began to speak for themselves and not negatively about each other.

Sonja commented very early on that on one occasion, Peter had turned beet red and had declared in vehement tones, "You shrew, you're always so suspicious of me!" Sonja picked up the language of the mediation therapist, asking Peter to put that accusation in the form of a request. He responded "Please, will you refrain from sharing your fears with me just as I am about ready to leave to meet my friends?" In so doing, Peter asked his wife to give him the benefit of the doubt. He asked her to assume that he is not sneaking around. He declared he had never and would never be unfaithful in this or any marriage, no matter how controlling she became: he would simply leave, as he had.

Sonja acknowledged that, in her head, she believed her

husband is and will be faithful to her. She acknowledged that she herself has a great deal of work to do on an emotional, visceral level to catch up with what her head knows to be true. She pointed out to her husband, however, that his leaving, experienced by her as abandonment, was not much better a prospect for her than his being unfaithful.

On his part, Peter's anger penetrated so deeply that it took him a considerable amount of time (much longer than it had taken Sonja) to acknowledge anything she had said. Initially, he would shake his head and look bitterly away when she spoke. It was noticeable when he said one day, "I know what you're saying, Sonja."

Very early on in the mediation therapy, the therapist addressed the asymmetry in the volume of their communication. Sonja initially appeared traumatized by the degree of rage she felt at having been left; she was unable to speak. (Far more typical is a wife who talks nonstop, with a husband furious on the sidelines.) The mediation therapist repeatedly told Peter and Sonja how very important it is for them to speak equally—for the sake of mutuality, symmetry, and neutrality. In this case, the therapist actually stopped Peter many times to obtain an equivalent communication from Sonja.

To this end, employing the rational structures from chapter 4 is useful, since they require a straightforward answer from each member of the couple. For example, when asked the question, "What did your partner bring to your unit, which you felt you lacked?" Peter mused that the same thing that bothers him so much now, Sonja's controllingness, seemed like the directiveness she had when he met her, which he so lacked initially. "If every sword has two edges, just make sure this one is lying with the directiveness side, not the controlling side, on top," remarked the mediation therapist.

As nearly every other couple does, the Andrews needed anger instruction. They labeled Sonja the angry one since she expressed her anger externally by yelling, throwing things— once even a whole

frozen chicken. The couple polarized, by labeling her the angry one and him the quiet

one; however, they were simply what Jurg Willi calls "polar variants" on the same

theme.[10] Peter internalized his anger, avoiding overt expression until he

could no longer stand it, then walking out of the marriage entirely, a very angry

expression.

In learning the two-step process of anger expression discussed previously, first

toxic-affective release, then more effective expression, Peter borrowed moderately

from his wife's direct expression for his first stage, expressing more physically and

verbally, while Sonja modeled herself on his ability to hold back on the extreme overt

expression of anger for her second stage. The two polar variants then met somewhere

in the middle by more effectively expressing angry feelings verbally. Sonja learned

particularly well the technique of visualizing having feelings such as jealousy or fear

of being abandoned without letting them consume her, so that she no longer became

those

feelings. She voiced pride in her new ability to keep her feelings in proper proportion.

Through a joint process of brainstorming options, Peter and Sonja and the mediation therapist devised a process of internal stroking, of gaining good feelings and self-praise when either of them successfully dealt with feelings that had previously been destructive. Sonja and her husband agreed that, initially, when she omitted sharing a jealous thought, with attendant good feeling, she could purchase an additional piece of her favorite antique stemware as she acquired a number of these omissions. And, initially, when Peter was able to identify a statement from his wife such as "Mr. G. certainly did give you a terrible haircut" as being one of having his best interests in mind, he similarly rewarded himself with good feelings, which were noted and led to his acquiring favorite household tools over a period of time.

During the mediation therapy process, Peter and Sonja had to journey to the Pacific Northwest to help care for Peter's elderly father. In the past, Sonja had been very uncomfortable staying in his parents' home because of some of the side effects of the elderly Mr. Andrews's disease. She was able to use techniques she had learned in negotiation instruction to bargain with Peter to stay with other relatives part of the time. He negotiated with Sonja to come with him, even though the future duration of their relationship was unknown.

Over the course of the mediation therapy, there were noticeable changes in the Andrews' behavior and communication. Both Sonja and Peter were able to quickly put aside needing to be right or wrong. They were thoroughly accustomed to blaming and accusing, but quickly began to say, for example, "I don't see it the way you do" and "I feel that my integrity is being questioned when you are suspicious of me."

As has been mentioned, Sonja and Peter came from radically different family and cultural backgrounds. In Peter's family conflict was expressed by acting out, by somatization, or not at all, and in Sonja's family conflict was dramatically expressed, then resolved, not by negotiation but by kissing and making up with dramatic resolutions never to fight again. To witness Peter and Sonja heatedly, skillfully, negotiating a difference, without any of the prior paroxysms of rage or walking away, was rewarding for the mediation therapist. The final and most rewarding witnessing by the mediation therapist was being in attendance while the Andrews negotiated returning to live with one another. They remain together today, with their three sons, their mediation therapy having taken place well over ten years ago.

Conclusion:
Negotiating Requires Two Unmerged Partners

The use of conflict negotiation techniques involves both intervention in the couple's conflict before they even come to the office, and teaching them assertive communication skills, conflict negotiation attitudes, and conflict negotiation techniques.

Structures or questions, which help the couple see themselves more clearly, help couples obtain the distance needed for resolution of conflicts. These techniques, designed to help people build bridges to one another, inevitably throw people back upon themselves in self-discovery. The road to the other inevitably involves finding the path to the self. Conflict between people and disturbance in a relationship may be seen as partially stemming from individuals' not taking responsibility for themselves, from their blaming the other for not providing what the self needs to provide.

Standing by while people learn to negotiate conflict is to witness individuals' taking themselves back as separate entities, entities that require separateness before they may ever negotiate a oneness or a further separateness for continuing growth. The essence of helping people to pragmatically resolve their interpersonal conflict is to aid them in ensuring that there are not one but two distinct parties to the conflict.

Notes

[1] Fisher and Ury, *Getting to Yes*, 23.

[2] Bernard, *Conflict Resolution with a Couple*.

[3] Ibid.

[4] Gorman, Ira, "Decision Making Workshop"

[5] Dawes, 227.

[6] Fisher and Ury, *Getting to Yes*, 131.

[7] Ibid

[8] Bernard

[9] Ibid, 32..

[10] Willi, Couples in Collusion, 56.

Decision Making

At a midpoint in the mediation therapy process, the mediation therapist will express her or his confidence in each individual's ability to eventually integrate rational, sensory, emotional, intuitive, and instructional information into an inner knowing. It is my belief that decision making about relationships is not wholly rational, or even primarily rational. It is with courage that people leap to the knowledge of their decisions, looking backward in an effort to define how and why they know what they know. "I just know." "Now I *understand*." "It is clear as a bell to me, now." These are all expressions of reaching the culmination of the decision making.

As has been said previously, in attempting to make a decision, people frequently look as though they have an adding machine tape behind opaque eyes, the tape emerges from either side of their heads, one side with yes written on it, the other with no written on it. Their eyes move back and forth from one side to the other in an attempt to make a decision. This sashaying, cognitively, from one side of the conflict to the other is painful to watch and employs only one of many faculties for decision making.

Often each side of the conflict, if chosen, represents choices individuals don't seem willing to live with. What is frequently needed, instead of an external choice, is an internal shift in understanding in the conflicted party. If decision making is not best described as a back and forth look between the choices, in what ways can it be described better?

A Metaphor for Decision Making

My own metaphor for decision making is the aforementioned metaphor embodied in the 1989 film *Field of Dreams*: if one builds a field, a desired resolution will take place. On the field (that is, in the mediation therapy process) is planted rational understanding, sensory and instructional information, intuition, emotional and inner wisdom. Cognitive rumination is not planted on the field, only cognitive understanding. The mediation therapist tends the field with basic conflict negotiation attitudes and techniques. When the time is right, a decision with a sense of integrated understanding will grow up on the field—that is, in the human heart, gut, or inner self.

My own image for a decision is a corn plant—not particularly aesthetic, but sturdy, alive, and sustaining. (Coincidentally, Barbara McClintoch, a researcher mentioned in *Women's Ways of Knowing*, who won the Nobel Prize for work on the genetics of corn plants, wrote that you have to have patience "to hear what [the corn] has to say to you" and the openness "to let it come to you."[1]) In my image, when the corn plant is full grown on the field, a person has been patient enough to gather all the information from within and without to understand exactly what the corn plant is saying to him or her. Each individual using the *Field of Dreams* making will create his or her own image for the decision he or she is making.

The mediation therapy evokes a wealth of information, which is planted in individuals in whom a decision will grow. They will not have to ruminate about the decision, or figure it out in their heads. The mediation therapy decision makers frequently look peaceful and calm during the intervention. They have made a decision not to foreclose on an eventual decision without the necessary information. They have their eyes, their ears, and their feelings wide open and are receptive to their intuition and to their inner wisdom. They have suspended a frantic search for an immediate decision. They have trust that they can endure a period of not knowing in order to arrive at silent knowledge or inner knowing. They are told that they will be able to blend a wide variety of information—multiple variables—into the making of a decision. Frequently the structured decision-making process will help frightened individuals engage some calmness and serenity within themselves.

In a workshop on decision making, Ira Gorman explains that "much of human thought is automatic. People reach conclusions by following chains of associations. Although decisions have multiple implications, decision makers usually pay attention to one or possibly two variables to the exclusion of other important ones. The process of thinking automatically and limiting the number of variables is usually adaptive in a world in which we are flooded with information. We simply couldn't function if we paid attention to everything." The goal of Gorman's decision making workshop is "to help people go beyond automatic thinking when they have important decisions to make. [Individuals] learn to weigh multiple considerations, generate new options, and be open to new information so that they can see decisions sooner and start to think and act when it is possible for them to have maximum impact."[2] Being open to a wealth of new information through all of the structures in mediation therapy; creating new options through brainstorming

—

and negotiation skills; and weighing many more decisions than the mind typically holds, are all integral to the decision-making process in mediation therapy.

Making a decision involves letting go of the familiar. People know the status quo, how things are. A decision typically involves change, something new. Change is frequently resisted, even when it results in a positive outcome. Where decisions entail the possibility of change, resistance is not far behind. Even if the current situation is miserable, it is familiar.

As previously discussed, asking what the positives are in the current situation is one way to address resistance to decision making. The couple mentioned earlier who fought incessantly said that the good part of the way things were in their relationship for him was that he was able to preserve a sense of space and independence; for her it was the ability to maintain her own identity, which she had been unable to do in her first marriage. Acknowledging with the couple the positives in their fighting may have given them permission to somehow say to themselves, "The positives are good, but they aren't all there is to it; we pay a huge price for those positives of space and identity."

Another strategy for getting through resistance to decision making is asking *why* making a decision is a bad idea. Typical answers are:

"We will have to do something different." "There will

be no turning back."
"We lose options when we choose one option."

If making a decision, then, truly seems to be a bad idea, then the non-decision makers at least understand why they are not making a decision.

In the reverse, asking why an individual wants to make a

decision brings to the fore the desires to finally get out of a limbo state, to put an end

to confusion, to get started in a forward direction. Even though arriving at a decision

is experienced as difficult, even painful, realizing the positives in doing so may give

the decision makers added courage.

Inner Knowing

Around session seven or eight, the mediation therapist, in an aside, might mention

that she or he sees decision making as gradually accumulating new information,

weighing many considerations, and creating new options. Once this rational

information has been assimilated, individuals may move rapidly and intuitively to a

conclusion. If the rational processes are like roads down which the cognitive

processes travel, and the conscious mind like a fallow field that is seeded by the

answers to the rational structures, as well as by sensory information, emotional

sharing and by education, then the decision is like a strong plant that grows up in the

field, surrounded perhaps by

little wildflowers or tentative answers or conclusions. This image, and other statements made along the way about decision making, is intended to help people relax and trust in the knowledge that they are indeed *doing* the decision-making work, some linear, some nonlinear, and that the decision will spring from the accumulation of their work. Theodore Isaac Rubin talks about "integrated concentration" as "bringing our total selves— all our resources, time and energy— into focus on the action at hand, to the exclusion of all other matters. If it accompanies the carrying out of a decision, it is an enormously powerful and effective force."[3]

—

During sessions eight to ten of a twelve-session contract, I ask individuals (as does family therapist Sallyann Roth) to take their partner's position on the question at hand, speaking to and arguing for that position as if it were their own.[4] The partner's position may then be experienced as more objective, as more free- floating than being seen as wedded to the partner. Taking one another's positions can be done repeatedly, and may result in freeing solidly entrenched positions and in experiencing ambivalence about the decision. A newly ambivalent state may contribute to a person's eventually moving back to an original position, or moving to the possibility of blending both partners' decisions, or even in moving toward agreement with the partner's position. Ambivalence allows the freeing up of solid, static positions.

Distinguishing between making or figuring out a decision cognitively and uncovering a decision that has been growing within and has been well fertilized by the mediation therapy process, is important. Not looking back and forth frantically between options, but trusting, waiting, learning, then leaping with courage to a decision is the mode presented in mediation therapy.

Toward session nine, the mediation therapist will say, "Soon, you each will be able to make your decision without using words. Some people know their decisions in their hearts, others in their guts or in their essential selves or beings." Telling people they will be able to know is highly effective. In *Mindfulness* Ellen Langer says, "Keeping free of mindsets, even for a moment, we may be able to see clearly and deeply."[5] All of the suggestions of the mediation therapist to tune in to inner knowing, and to clear the mind of rational inquiry, in order to see clearly, are like Langer's suggestion that "In an intuitive or mindful state, new information, like new melodies, is allowed into awareness."[6] The new information fertilizes the fallow fields so that a decision may grow up and be discovered. Henri Poincare said it well: "It is by logic that we prove. It is by intuition that we discover."[7] The predominant message to our clients is to get out of their own ways; to have trust in their own rich processes of gathering data (sensory, rational, emotional, educational information) and synthesizing this data into committed, self-connected decisions.

Reconnecting to information that people have screened out, in order to support the status quo, may cause people considerable discomfort. Recognizing a new decision may result in people feeling foolish or wrongheaded about their past decisions. When this occurs I often explain that, faced with a series of alternatives, people make decisions that have certain gains and certain prices. At a later time, the price may well outweigh the gain. The original decision, however, may have been the best decision available from the alternatives at the time. Because a new decision is currently seen as more appropriate, does not mean that an old decision in its time was in error.

Decision making is clearly a process, not an event. Instruction about decision making is not done of a piece, but in discrete enjoinders throughout:

"The combination of all you are learning will yield
creative decisions."

"The seeds for your decision are within you."

"How would you feel if you did know what direction to
take with your relationship?"

"If you knew your decision, what would it be?" "Do you know anyone who knows how to decide?" "What stops you from trusting your inner resources?" At times, I will read from Carlos Castenada's The Power of Silence:

> I am just considering how our rationality puts us between a rock and a hard place. Our tendency is to ponder, to question, to find out. And there is no way to do that .... Reaching the place of silent knowledge cannot be reasoned out. It can only be experienced. So close the door of self-reflection. Be impeccable and you'll have the energy to reach the place of silent knowledge.[8]

I say that when people know their decisions from silent or inner knowledge, they may be able to look backward, through all the information they have gathered, to understand how and why they know what they know. To quote Castenada again, "Man's predicament is that he intuits his inner resources, but he does not use them."[9]

—

It must be clear by this time that I believe that many people in this culture have the illusion that mind or rational senses are what make decisions, that "Conscious mind is too damn cocky," as Bandler and Grinder put it.[10] Students in classes of mediation therapy have shared that their important decisions have been processes, not rational conclusions. The above instruction—to merely *include* rational understanding in decision making—is interwoven with instruction that mutual decision making or mutually understood decision making cuts down on one partner's assuming all the guilt, while the other assumes a victim position. Common sense shows that unilateral decision making results in less well-being for partners and children than mutually made, or at least mutually understood, decisions.

Prior to asking for individual decisions about the future direction of the relationship (or another decision), the mediation therapist may make some statement such as:

> You certainly have a great deal more information to use as a basis
> for making decisions; you have been considerate of your

children's needs during this time of indecision; you've learned new skills of assertiveness, communication, negotiation, disagreement, and decision making. With all these inputs, I believe you can trust yourself to leap, with courage, to a decision, to inner knowing, perhaps only looking back later to understand the decision. May you now move out of the impasse of anger, sadness, stuckness, or immobility to a position where you are able to perceive an inner decision.

Of course, the statement should be tailor-made by the individual mediation therapist. Another example might be:

You most likely see yourself, your partner, and your relationship more clearly now. I hope you have come to trust your intuition, that you have asked and been granted forgiveness and have forgiven your partner what was important to forgive. You are, I believe, ready to know your decision.

Unlike the more explicit rational structures, assistance in decision making through inner knowing is more subtle instructional work resulting in attitudinal and belief shifts which are less visible than overt changes in behavior.

Rational Decision Making

Harold Greenwald in *Decision Therapy* has summarized his

ideas, which may be used as part of the rational decision-making process from session six to twelve:

1. State your problem as clearly and completely as you can.

2. Examine past decisions that helped create the problem.

3. List the payoffs for the past decisions that are behind the problem.

4. Answer the question: what was the context in which you made the original decision?

5. Examine alternatives to your past decision. 6. Choose your alternative and put it into practice.[11] Mediation therapists who attempt Greenwald's six-question model for themselves will understand the usefulness of the decision-making questions. People accustomed to using decision trees might benefit from such an analysis, especially when indecisiveness has taken over.

Robin Dawes in *Rational Choice in An Uncertain World* presents an arithmetic method of assigning numerical weights to choices.[12] For people who enjoy numbers and who are stuck in the decision-making process, Dawes' approach may be the wrench which unscrews the stuck nut of indecision.

Max Bazerman in *Judgment in Managerial Decision Making* describes a six step "rational" decision-making process which mediation therapists may want to incorporate into the rational structures. Bazerman's six steps are:

7. Define the problem

8. Identify the criteria (or objectives) 9. Weight

the criteria
10. Generate alternatives

11. Rate each alternative on each criterion 12. Compute

the optimal decision[13]

In mediation therapy the problem is accurately defined as the need and desire to reach a decision. Often, the criteria or objectives for a couple in reaching a decision are to get themselves out of limbo and pain; to become more attentive parents; and to move forward with their lives. Couples know the relative value of their objectives. With the assistance of the mediation therapist, couples identify as many courses of action as they can, seeing how well each alternative solution achieves each of their criteria or objectives. In mediation therapy, what Bazerman calls "computing the optimal decision" could include his elaborate prescription for computation and/or factoring in the above steps along with sensory, emotional, intuitive, and educational information.

The Decisions

It is a momentous time when individuals are asked for their decisions. Often people will have known a decision before the conclusion of mediation therapy. Sometimes decisions come as a complete surprise. Frequently people will acknowledge that it isn't the decision they want to make (in the case of divorce), but it is the decision they know is the right decision for all concerned. A lot of pain may well be experienced frequently at this point, as well as relief that a decision has been made. Each individual will be helped to clarify how he or she regards and feels about the decision. Each will be helped to be comfortable with the decision, however painful. Often, the essence of Theodore Isaac Rubin's following statement is conveyed to clients: "Working at decision-making means taking advantage of the human prerogative. We alone, as a species have the potential of choice and decision—of options beyond instinctual, biological dictates. This is real freedom. This is real power. Making decisions gives us the freedom to exert power in living our own lives."[14]

———

The critical final step in mediation therapy is to help the partners negotiate their integrated individual decisions to a mutually acceptable or, at least, mutually understood decision. If both individuals have decided to be further committed to the relationship on an ongoing basis and want to work with a professional or professionals to enhance their relationship, the mediation therapist may provide them with referrals or entertain their request to work with the mediation therapist in a new capacity, after a break in time. If the individuals have both decided to divorce, assessment of their children's needs and their own ongoing personal and legal/mediation needs is in order. If one partner has decided to commit to the relationship and the other clearly wants out, sometimes all that can be done, as stated earlier, is that the partner who wants the marriage goes on record as being in opposition to the divorce. Hopefully, he or she can state why the other finds it necessary to dissolve their union, can understand at minimum, why something so painful is necessary from the partner's point of view. More than occasionally a partner will not want to leave a marriage but will say that under the circumstances he or she also desires a divorce, since a marriage involves two people who want it.

In the negotiation of individual decisions, I strive for the highest level of agreement or understanding possible between partners. Certainly angry feelings are legitimate at this stage and help the couple disengage from one another. The anger may coexist with an attempt, at least, to understand the partner's need for such a drastic decision.

Once people have reached the highest level of agreement and understanding possible at this point, plans to implement their decision are begun. Getting to those decisions involves men and women learning to respect and integrate their own rational, emotional, sensory, and intuitive knowledge into what Castenada might agree could be described as "the somersault of thought into the inconceivable."[15]

—

Notes

[1] Belenky, et at. 143.

[2] Gorman, "Decision Making Workshop."

[3] Rubin, Overcoming Indecisiveness, 181.

[4] Roth, "Designing Tasks That Help Couples Continue Their Therapy At Home" lecture.

[5] Langer, Mindfulness, 118.

[6] Ibid., p.118

[7] Henri Poincare, "Intuition and Logic Mathematics," 205-212.

[8] Castendada, The Power of Silence, 87.

[9] Ibid., 249

[10] Bandler and Grinder, *Frogs into Princes*, 185.

[11] Rubin, 204.

[12] Greenwald, Decision Therapy, 299.

[13] Bazerman, Judgment in Managerial Decision Making, 3-4.

[14] Dawes, 227.

[15] Castenada, 132.

Children's Needs

The child's efforts at mastery are strengthened when he understands the divorce as a serious and carefully considered remedy for an important problem, when the divorce appears purposeful and rationally undertaken, and indeed succeeds in bringing relief and a happier outcome for one or both parents.

—Judith S. Wallerstein and Joan Berlin Kelly, *Surviving the*

Breakups[1]

AT THE TIME parents raise concerns about their children, or at the time they have decided on a marital separation or divorce, it is appropriate to share information about children's needs with a couple. I often ask them if they believe there is such a thing as a healthy adjustment for children of divorce. And if there is in their hearts and minds a healthy adjustment, is there one living arrangement for the children that they believe to be better than others? Is living primarily with one parent, and visiting the other, or living equally or part of the time with each parent a better arrangement? One hopes that helping them be in touch with their biases about children's adjustments and living arrangements liberates them to listen to what you have to say about research findings and your own experience. Once they know they have biases and what they are, they are more apt to listen to you talk about your observations, experience, and research findings, rather than screening out what you are saying because it disagrees with what they believe.

Living Arrangements After Divorce

An excellent point of departure for helping parents to create appropriate postdivorce living arrangements is to brainstorm together with the mediation therapist the qualities of parenting that can make a difference in the adjustment of their children. When parents derive for themselves what their children will need, I sense that the parents will honor those requirements.

With regard to living arrangements after divorce, I indicate that I believe there are several living arrangements in which children prosper after divorce, depending upon factors such as the children's ages, temperaments, gender, and vulnerability toward experiencing loyalty conflicts between parents. Fortunately—or unfortunately, according to one's viewpoint—there seem to be no magic formulas, no rules that say all children are better off living with one parent and visiting the other, or better off living with each parent part of the time.

It is reported in Wallerstein and Blakeslees' book *Second Chances: Men, Women and Children after Divorce, Who Wins, Who Loses—and Why* [by Judith S. Wallerstein and Sandra Blakeslee, New York: Ticknor & Fields, 1989] that quality of parenting, cooperation between parents, and settling of conflicts between the two parents are important issues in children's adjustment. I suggest these issues may be even more important than the number of homes in which the children live. I tell parents that it will not be possible to sit in their lawyer's or divorce mediator's office and design a living arrangement schedule that will guarantee adjustment and happiness for children. I tell them that, in my view, the task is infinitely more difficult than deciding where the children reside. It involves parents *being with their children*, sustaining a quality relationship with them consistently over a long period of time. It involves learning new parenting skills, and, as Wallerstein indicates, making the children a *major* priority.

Separating or divorcing parents cannot design the structure of the house—the living arrangements for the children— neglecting what goes on *within* the house for the next eight or fifteen or twenty years. In choosing which postdivorce parenting arrangement is the best for each couple, I say that, in eighteen years as a family psychotherapist and eleven years as a divorce and family mediator, I have learned for myself that the chief factor in choosing a parenting arrangement, after divorce, is a realistic assessment of what the capacities and limitations are in the parenting relationship between two good people. Table 8-1 delineates factors that, in my experience, may lead to a good outcome and those that may lead to a poor outcome for children of divorce.

Collaborative/Cooperative Mode

In the early 1990s, conventional wisdom's ideal postdivorce

parenting   arrangement   seems   the
                                                        to   be

collaborative/cooperative mode, which often mirrors a joint legal custody decision,

and presumes that the couple has the ability to make cooperative decisions in areas of

the children's medical, educational, and religious needs.

I tell people that it takes two individuals who are truly *capable* of collaboration, not

just *willing* to collaborate. I ask that each assess his or her own and the other's ability

to be genuinely cooperative, including considering travel time away from the area in

which the children reside, geographical and emotional distance from one another any

workaholism, alcoholism, and so forth. Is each of them—in terms of temperament,

and by virtue of career- stage, remarriage, level of anger or antagonism—

capable of and truly desirous of a collaborative parenting arrangement?

If people believe that they *must* be capable, by virtue of contemporary trend and desire, but find themselves falling short each time they attempt to collaborate, their individual selfesteem will most likely be decreased rather than enhanced, by virtue of having selected a postdivorce parenting arrangement that they are not in actual fact capable of carrying out.

I tell people that admitting to themselves that this mode is not for them or is not working, is ceasing to fail every single time they do not achieve collaboration. They may feel like failures in not achieving an ideal, like women who attempt natural childbirth, but need medication, or women who would like to nurse their babies and cannot in practice do so. In both cases the better part of wisdom says to accept reality, not trying to do battle for the sake of an ideal. People may always reassess their assumptions and agreements about what they thought they were capable of doing—the sections of divorce agreements having to do with the children may be modified.

Tandem Mode

I tell people that if collaborative/cooperative postdivorce parenting arrangements aren't for them, for whatever reason, they may still have joint legal custody or joint decision making by choosing, on their own, what I call a *tandem*, separate but equal arrangement of parenting. In this mode, each parent is capable of assuming one hundred percent of the responsibility for each child. Each parent puts parenting very high on his or her list of priorities. These parents, however, don't often do well or enjoy conferring frequently with one another about anything. They elect to meet infrequently and often with a third party present, to discuss important aspects of the children's rules, discipline, material and emotional needs, their scheduling, and so forth. These parents should pledge to be as civil as possible for the sake of their children, writing to one another when necessary and conferring in person when that is required. They should pledge

especially not to send their children back and forth with messages from one another.

They will not want to make their inabilities to confer into a burden for their children

by asking them to be go-betweens.

In some cases, one parent, often a mother but more and more frequently a father;

will have an uneven amount of responsibility for the children. *Quality* of parenting

by both parents is the important ingredient. Minimizing the transitions and the

disruptions that accompany the transitions is an asset of this mode. Parents may, of

course have joint decision making custody of the children, even though the amount of

time they actually spend with the children is unequal or uneven. The parent who has

less time with the children may be in frequent telephone contact with the children,

keep the postal carrier busy, as well as have a close relationship with the teacher

and principal at the children's school whether near or far from his or her residence.

Even where there is antagonism between parents,

the school where the child spends the majority of his or her waking hours during the school year, may well be a neutral place where both parents can track their children's social, academic, and emotional growth.

I tell people about the two-year-old boy whose mother had no understanding of the continuing importance of his contact with his father. Rather than moving some distance away to be near her family, she took the mediation therapist's information about children's needs to heart and decided to stay near the father. He in turn has called the boy every night for three years to say goodnight; he also takes his son two evenings a week for dinner and one overnight a week. The boy lives primarily with his mother, but has by no means lost his dad. The two parents can barely stand the sight of one another but are trying hard not to cripple their son with their antipathy. The little boy, by all reports, is flourishing.

Single/Predominantly Single Mode

The last postdivorce parenting mode I mention is the single or predominantly single style, the advantages of which are the ease involved when one need not coordinate, check things out with, or plan with the other parent. The disadvantages are that children lack enough contact with and input from the other parent, and, in addition, the parenting parent is not getting help from, relief by, or coordination with another parent. This mode should be chosen when a parent is dangerous to a child— physically or sexually abusive, or having an acute or chronic untreated mental illness, for example. This mode will benefit those children who need to be separated from the abuse or the illness. Sole legal custody would be the most likely form of legal decision making chosen for this type of parenting arrangement. Table 8-2 illustrates the correlation between styles of parenting, actual living arrangements of children, and legal custody options.

Regardless of which mode parents choose for parenting during marital separation and divorce, both parents will need to learn new skills. Some will need to learn to set consistent, firm limits, some will need to learn to nurture, to listen, to be on duty constantly. It won't do to say, "Oh well, they are allowed to stay up indefinitely at the other house; it must be part of their character by now ... I won't need to enforce bedtime here either," or, "They travel so much with the other parent, I better travel equally with them, as well."

When people in mediation therapy choose to separate or divorce, I frequently will share my belief that, at least as important as their marriage vows were, and probably more so, are the vows they make to their children at this time. These vows may be individual and private, or collective and shared with the children. In any event, they are serious vows and tailored to meet the kinds of commitments parents want and need to make to their children at this time. I give two sorts of vows as examples:

A mother's vow to her teenage son might be:

I willingly take responsibility, to the best of my ability, for nurturing your growth and development. I will not wait for your father to keep you in line, to set those firm limits for you, but will do so myself. I promise that I will not do too many things for you, because it is easier for me, but will foster your doing for yourself, for your self-confidence, and competence. When I cannot provide for your needs, I promise to get the kind of help for you or myself that I believe we need. I choose not to feel or act like a victim, a "poor me" mother left with the care of a teen-age boy, but to feel and act like a mature, autonomous, and responsible parent, who is very proud to be your mother.

The parents of three young children might vow:

If it were not vitally necessary, and if we hadn't given it years of thought, we—your parents—would not choose to live in two different homes. Since it has become necessary to do so, we pledge to continue to communicate weekly about you, and more often, if necessary. We will talk about how you are doing with the new living arrangements, in school and outside of school. We intend to be present for you, together as your parents when appropriate: at your ballgames, skating shows, graduations, weddings, the births of your children. We intend not to spoil you, but to see that your emotional, your physical, and your spiritual needs will be met to the best of our abilities.

Research Findings

How can we, as mediation therapists, use the research that has been done on the effects of divorce on children to help parting parents keep their vows to their children? For one thing, we can avoid taking research too literally. Knowing findings of research studies is like having a chart of a large lake. The shortest distance from point A to point B on the chart may appear to be to go due east yet the chart doesn't provide information on prevailing winds, or daily weather patterns. To illustrate, a psychologist called me to ask what research findings indicate about the preferred living arrangements for four-yearold girls. The psychologist's clients were calling to ask whether their four-year-old daughter should live in two homes (Sunday to Wednesday in one house and after school Wednesday to afternoon Sunday in the other, rather than living with Mom and visiting Dad every weekend, with an overnight every other weekend). What guidance can any helping professional provide?

Susan Steinman's research project on joint custody showed that many four- and five-year-old girls, and some seven- and eight-year-old boys experienced confusion about which home they were going home to at any given time.[2] And Wallerstein's research, reported in *Second Chances,* showed some evidence that elementary school children can handle time, distance, and alternating schedules more effectively than can pre-school children.[3] Are these two pieces of evidence enough to advise the couple to have their daughter live in one home, primarily?

What about evidence that fathers stay better involved and are themselves less depressed when they have more access to their children? Is this an important consideration? This couple wondered whether they should discount their individual needs as a two-career divorcing couple: each needed time without their daughter to attend to the myriad of administrative details of running a home alone, to say nothing of time needed to establish themselves socially as independent entities. These parents were delighted to know about some research relative to their daughter's needs, and they realized they needed to be aware of their specific child's personality and special needs, as well as their own needs. They decided to have their daughter live with each of them part of the week, graduating to a whole week at a time later on, and then two weeks at a later time as she grows older. Their daughter's input along the way would be solicited and given the greatest of consideration. They decided that for the time being, she would wear red sneakers while at Mom's house and blue while at Dad's home. They intend to be in close communication with her preschool teachers and principal, who are aware that they desire her well-being, above their own convenience or needs. They explicitly asked school personnel how their parenting arrangements appear to be affecting their daughter. They were willing to change arrangements as many times as necessary and so indicated. They heard information about transitions being difficult for children, and spoke of the once per week transition at midweek being less of a disruption than two at the beginning and end of every weekend, with a probable third and fourth if Dad took his daughter for dinner twice a week, which he would want to do, rather than waiting until the weekend to see her. Research, I tell people, should be used as a guideline to inform one's own notions of what would be the best solution for a particular child.

As a mediation therapist, I have highlighted or selectively noted aspects of research on joint custody and on the effects of divorce on children and parents. I share this information with my clients both in chart form (see charts at the end of this chapter) and verbally.

Stresses and Benefits of Children Living in Two Homes

Steinman's Study. Susan Steinman's small research project on joint custody reported in 1981 delineates stresses and benefits of living in two homes at least 33 percent of the time with each parent; some aspects of her research that I find helpful are presented in the following lists.[4]

Steinman lists the following as stresses:

Where parents were in conflict over child-rearing values,

there were troubled kids. [I believe this may be so, regardless of the number of homes in which the children reside.]

Where one parent was financially or emotionally less well-off than the other, there were worried kids.

One-third of all kids in the study had loyalty conflicts. One girl commented that it could never be equal between her parents because there were seven days in the week. Another had to remember to give Dad a kiss if she had kissed Mom.

One-fourth of all kids (including one-half of all four- to five-years old girls and many seven- to eight-yearold boys) experienced confusion about which home they were to be in, when.

Distance between homes was a problem for some children, but not for others.

Many adolescents demonstrate needing increased control over their lives and the loosening of psychological ties to their parents.

Even though they knew it wasn't feasible, most of the kids

wished their parents were back together again.

One-third of the children felt *overburdened by maintaining*
a strong presence in two homes [emphasis added].

In all families in the study, maintaining two households
required considerable effort on the parts of parents and
children, alike.

On the other hand, Steinman's study found several benefits of two homes:

Having two involved parents to whom they were strongly
attached. They did not suffer feelings of rejection or abandonment
often seen in children whose non-custodial parent does not maintain
frequent and regular contact.

Their sense of importance in their family—that their
parent had gone to a great deal of effort to maintain the joint
custody—and this enhanced their sense of self-esteem. They felt wanted by
both parents.

Most of the children were not torn by loyalty conflicts, but rather felt free to love and be with both parents.[5] **Wallerstein's Studies.**

I find many of Judith Wallerstein's findings about children living in two homes—with joint physical custody—salient for the mediation therapy population. Dr. Wallerstein reports that the overall quality of life and the relationships between members of a family are what determine the well-being of children of divorce. The joint custody research indicates that the frequency of transitions between households could be upsetting to children. Wallerstein's findings show that two years after divorce, children raised in joint custody households—that is, children who live in two households with either parent—are no better adjusted than children raised in sole custody households. By itself, after two years, joint custody does not minimize the negative impact of divorce on children. Over a longer period of time, Wallerstein suggests joint custody may have positive psychological effects[6].

The mediation therapist is likely to benefit by knowing about Wallerstein's proposal of additional psychological tasks that children of divorce need to accomplish in addition to the normal developmental

tasks[7]. Seven tasks are listed and described below:

· understanding the divorce ·

strategic withdrawal · dealing with

loss · dealing with anger · working

out guilt

· accepting the permanence of the divorce · taking a

chance on love

Understanding the divorce is described by Wallerstein as achieving a realistic

understanding of what divorce means in the child's family, along with the concrete

consequences of divorce for a particular child. I tell mediation therapy clients that

their children need to acknowledge the reality of the household changes, and, as Wallerstein says, they need to differentiate their fantasy fears from reality.

Strategic withdrawal means that as they divorce and live separately, parents need to understand that their children will benefit by disengaging from parental conflict and stress, resuming their customary social and academic pursuits. Wallerstein emphasizes that children need their parents' support to remain children.

The task of absorbing loss is described by Wallerstein as the most difficult task imposed on children by divorce. Children are required to "overcome the profound sense of rejection, humiliation, vulnerability and powerlessness they feel with the departure of one parent. When the parent leaves, children of all ages blame themselves."[8] I tell mediation therapy clients that their children will need parental support and may need the support of professional psychotherapists, to grapple with and resolve multiple feelings of loss:

· the loss of the family unit and of self-identity as a member of the unit

· the loss of the presence of both parents together

· the possible loss of neighborhoods, schools, proximity of friends and relatives

Dealing with anger is a task that Wallerstein describes as difficult for children who feel both love and anger for parents whom they perceive as making attempts to improve their lives. I encourage parents to tell their children that they are able to accept their children's feelings about the divorce, including their intense feelings of anger and frustration.

Wallerstein indicates that the task of working out guilt for children implies going on with their own lives, untying themselves from the bond of guilt to a troubled parent. The task of accepting a divorce is done bit by bit by children, whose acceptance of the permanence of a divorce can not be achieved all at once.

Finally, the task of taking a chance on love requires the realistic assessment that while divorce is always a possibility in their own lives, young adults whose parents have divorced are capable of loving and being loved, of committing and of achieving fidelity[9].

—

Parents Talking with Children about Divorce

Predictably, in mediation therapy, soon after parents have made a decision to separate or divorce they wonder aloud about how to go about telling the children:

· when to tell them: right away, after their exams, when
    the school year ends, before or after they hear from colleges?

· whether to tell them as a unit, or the older ones together,
    the younger ones together or whether to tell them individually,
one-to-one? Should parents talk to children together or separately, or both?

· what to tell the children? Should all ages of children get

the same explanation?

Rather than giving definitive answers to these important questions, the mediation therapist sensitively explores the probable impact of various explanations of divorce, of timing, and of talking with various groupings of children. The mediation therapist eventually will come to have numerous alternative suggestions to add to the parents' own rational beliefs and intuitions about what, how, and when their children can hear about their decision to separate or to divorce.

Including Children in Mediation Therapy

The vast majority of parents in mediation therapy who choose to divorce are committed to attempting to minimize negative effects of divorce on their children. They are eager to learn information that will help them assist their children in remaining on track developmentally as much as possible. After a decision is made to separate or divorce, many parents ask for additional sessions to discuss their decision and its ramifications. Family groups with several teenage children virtually always request sessions with their children to discuss the decision. When a group of young adults clearly outnumbers the two parents, the parents seem to know instinctively that discussion with the mediation therapist as well as the children will facilitate the expression and resolution of feelings.

Teenagers and young adults want to ask various types of questions:

· What happened to the marriage?

· Are our parents okay? How is their mental health? · Will there be enough money to go around? · Will all of us still be able to go to college?

· Who will take on the departing parent's household responsibilities?

· How much time will we spend with each of our parents?

Parents sometimes opt to meet individually with some or each of their children. Particularly poignant are meetings between fathers and daughters, mothers and sons, where children ask parents tough questions, and parents give thoughtful, sensitive answers in spite of being in a great amount of pain. Individual meetings between one or two parents and a child, and group meetings of all children with the mediation therapist (or with their parents and the mediation therapist) are each effective in their own ways. Individual meetings provide children with the opportunity to ask pointed questions and provide parents with the opportunity to give information, reassurance and attention to a child individually. Group meetings seem to help young people collectively to express dissatisfactions with parents and with the situation. An eightyear-old girl and her father sobbed together about his leaving, while the mother and four-year-old daughter quietly shared in their grief. The relief and clear smiles on the faces of father, mother, and daughters after the session were indicators of the beginning of a transition from being stuck in inertia to the implementation of a

marital separation accomplished through a meeting of a whole family.

An example of an individual meeting between parent and child is a college-

age daughter who had the chance to express her sadness and intense anger with

her father who acknowledged that he was leaving the marriage for another woman.

The daughter ended the session by saying: "I love you very much, even though I am so

angry with you!"

Mediation therapists can be extraordinary resources for parents. They may convey

information about children's developmental needs at the time of divorce by

sharing experience, observations, and research findings about children, adolescents,

and young adults of divorce. Helping parents understand that their decision to

divorce has a potentially negative impact—as well as opportunities for growth—

is intended to help parents minimize negative impact on the

children and aid their children to grow through the experience. Through education and brainstorming, and by providing a forum in which parents and children together may face and discuss their mutual crisis, mediation therapists are part of a process of helping families plan for the future.

Summary

Each child is unique. Finding meaningful ways to talk with each child about the divorce, and to stay available to each of them for days after they are told about the decision, is important. Accurately recognizing each child's developmental stage and what that implies for her or his needs for reassurance and understanding is also important. In addition, each child's sadness, rage, anger, or disappointment is critical.

Perhaps even more important is that parents recognize their own feelings of desperation, fear of loneliness or of being abandoned and that they don't assume that their children feel this same way. Too frequently, through projective identification, parents falsely perceive in their children the sorrow or feelings of abandonment they are feeling themselves. In order to truly empathize with a child's feelings, a parent must be able to feel with the actual feelings of the child. A parent must try to hurt with him or her, without becoming the child, without taking over his or her feelings or assuming that the parents' own feelings belong to the child. A parent can be with the child, wherever he or she is, but the parent cannot make the feelings disappear, nor should he or she assume they are worse than they are. Accepting the child's own unique, separate feelings is the task at hand for divorcing parents. Being separate from the child is the only road to closeness.

Having made a carefully thought-out decision for separation or divorce in mediation therapy gives people a solid basis of inner conviction that they are taking the right course of action. This inner conviction has guided people in conveying to their children that they have made an important, well thought-out decision, which may unfortunately have negative impact on the whole family. Their convictions may help them convey as well that they care deeply about all of the children and intend to minimize the negative impact on all of them wherever possible.

Seeing themselves as people who want very much to make principled, well-considered decisions is part of the mediation therapy process. Although the road ahead, for children and parents alike, may be rocky in places, parents have every reason to believe that they will continue to act in the best interests of their children—trusting themselves to consider each individual's needs, just as they trusted themselves to make the best decision about the future direction of their relationship.

Notes

[1] Wallerstein and Kelly, 17

[2] .Steinman, 410.

[3] Wallerstein and Blakeslee, 268.

[4] Steinman, 403-414.

[5] Ibid.

[6] Wallerstein and Blakeslee, 270-272

[7] Ibid, 288-294.

[8] Ibid, 290.

[9] Ibid, 288-294.

Appendix:

Factors Influencing Adjustment of Children of Divorce

Table 8-1 Factors Determining Good versus Poor Outcome for Children of Divorce

These factors are derived from Miller Wiseman's eighteen years of working with and observing families in crisis and those separating and divorcing.

Factors for Parents to Consider Which May Facilitate a Good Outcome for Children of Divorce	Factors for Parents to Consider Which May Contribute to a Poor Outcome for Children of Divorce.
1. Making a thoughtful, well considered decision to separate or divorce.	1. The probable negative impact on children of parent suddenly being gone from the household.
2. Considering many alternative	2. The negative effect on

335

solutions to marriage crisis.

children of being given no (or an inadequate) explanation of the household rupture and no reassurance.

3. Sensitively informing children of the decision to divorce or separate, being aware of each child's developmental needs.

3. The negative effect on children of being given too many household responsibilities or too much responsibility for siblings or for parents' emotional stability.

4. Respecting each child's age appropriate need to maintain an internal mental and emotional image of each parent. Planning the frequency of parental contact around the child's need.

4. The negative impact on children of parents' taking over too many tasks for children or of over indulging children, due to their guilt about what children are undergoing.

5. Including the children, when appropriate, in the move from the household.

5. The negative impact of a parent choosing a child as a confidante or partner substitute.

6. The desirability of parents learning new ways to set limits and nurture in order to round out parenting skills.

6. The negative impact of a parent's being preoccupied with a new love, work, depression, anxiety, or unemployment.

7. The desirability of parents reinforcing each other's limit

7. The negative impact of a parent or a sibling being

setting with the children and not undermining one another.

8. The importance of parents being 8.
   predictably,

consistently there for their children.

9. The importance of parents 9.
   providing
appropriate, safe caregivers for children in their absence.

10. The importance of a realistic 10.
    assessment of each child's developmental

level; explanations

about the divorce, expectations of each child are geared to an ageappropriate level.

verbally, physically, or sexually

abusive or neglectful, consciously or unconsciously.

The negative impact of parents' undermining each others'

limitsetting, authority, or esteem.

The negative impact of excluding children from romantic or even platonic relationships of parents

The negative impact of an actual physical loss of one parent, or the emotional loss resulting from the neglect or illness of a parent.

Table 8-2 Styles of Postdivorce Parenting

Style	Requirements	Possible Living Arrangements	Legal Custody Typically	dy lly
Collaborative/ Cooperative Mode *Parents talk together*	Having the *ability* not just willingness to collaborate with other parent	Two homes Primary home with one parent; visitation by the	Joint	

Mode	Capacity	Living arrangement	Custody
		noncustodial parent in or out of the house Single home; other parent lives close by or at some distance	
Tandem Mode Capacity *Parents talk through a third party*	to assume responsibility for each child Ability to accept that frequent cooperation/collaboration with the other parent is not possible Meeting with or writing to other parents as often as necessary to communicate about children's needs Agreeing not to communicate by asking children to be go-betweens	Two homes Primary home with one parent; other parent visits, but not in the home.	Joint
Single/ Predominantly Single Mode *One parent is predominant*	Having the ability to parent with little or no input from the other parent	Children live in one home predominantly Other parent away; other parent not involved Other parent occasionally involved	Sole

Table 8-3

Talking with Children, Adolescents, and Young Adults About Divorce:
Developmental Stage Considerations

The complexity of the explanation of a divorce, depends upon many considerations, including children's ages and developmental stages. The following proposal in chart form consists of stagetypical principles for talking to children about divorce at various stages of their psychological development.

Principles for Talking with PreSchool Children about Divorce	Example of Principle
	Parent says to child:
	"It's not your fault that Mommy and Daddy aren't together, and you're not bad."
Parents help child:	
	"I know when you're with me you still love Mommy. Sometimes, you miss your mom a lot and you get a tummyache or headache. When that happens, let me know, and we'll call Mom."
• By helping child reduce self blame.	
• By helping child develop and maintain a secure internal mental-emotional image of both parents.	"Daddy is coming tonight and every Tuesday and Thursday to take you to dinner. And you will sleep over night at Dad's every weekend —all the green days we've marked on the calendar."
• By helping child to understand the concrete consequences of divorce for his or her own life.	"Daddy and I will make sure you have enough food, clothes, toys and love at both houses."
• By providing continuing physical care, love and support to each of their children.	

Principles for Talking with Elementary School Children	Example of Principle
Parents help child:	Parent says to child:
• By helping child reduce self blame.	"You are not at all to blame for the divorce. It's not your fault even though you might feel or think it's your fault. There's nothing you could have done differently."
• By reassuring child that attempts to divide parents, manipulate them, cause them to be competitive or antagonistic will not work.	"Telling me Dad lets you do it at his house won't work to get what you want at this house. "
• By reassuring child and demonstrating that she will not fall between the cracks, that parents will meet regularly to talk about their accomplishments and needs.	"Mom and I talk regularly about how you're doing and about what we both feel you need."
• By being open to child's reactions to divorce and by understanding that emotional reactions will be life-long and will reoccur with each developmental stage.	"I know it must be very hard and confusing to live in two different places with two sets of friends, two bedrooms, two neighborhoods." "You can count on me to pick you up every blue day on your calendar."
• By being consistent, not changing visitation plans, living arrangements suddenly. Schedules, colored charts will be made to make life more predictable for child.	
• By being prepared to give child	"Every Tuesday evening you can

one- to-one attention for several years after separation to attempt to ameliorate the losses.

• Minimize feeling pulled apart, caught in the middle, stretched to the breaking point.

• By attempting not to overindulge child with toys, food, vacations, sleeping with the child.

• By encouraging and helping the child talk about his or her feelings to appropriate others.

• By not encouraging child to be parent-like, taking on too much responsibility or by being a confidante to parents.

• By understanding child's regression in development initially after separation.

• By hearing child's wishes that parents reunite, explaining the reality, while sympathizing with the wish for reconciliation.

• By constantly demonstrating to the child that parents are consistent, reliable, predictable, still protective.

• By recognizing that if both parents suddenly need to work, the child will experience another loss—of a parent who is consistently at home.

count on just the two of us doing something special together."

"Sometimes kids feel they can't make everybody happy. When you feel this stress, let me know."

"I know that sometimes buying toys makes you feel better. I love you very much even though I'm not buying toys today."

"There are a lot of kids and even grownups who can understand your feelings."

"I appreciate your concern about my breaking up with Jim. How are you feeling about not having him around much any more?"

"I know it really hurts right now. Let's spend the whole morning doing just what you'd like to do."

"It's natural to want your parents back together again. I sympathize with wanting that, but it isn't going to happen."

"I just want you to know that wherever I'm living, I will try to be there for you in big and little emergencies as best I can."

"It's a BIG change to have your parents divorce and your Mom working at the same time. I know it's hard. What would make it better?"

Principles for Talking With Junior High School Children	Examples of Principle
Parents help child: • By reducing self-blame.	Parent says to child: "You didn't do anything to cause the divorce. The problems were between Mom and me."
• By reducing child's need to take on the role of the absent parent.	"I appreciate your doing the grocery shopping, but I want to be sure it isn't interfering with your homework and soccer."
• By encouraging child to share thoughts and feelings about the divorce with appropriate others.	"When you're ready, it can be helpful to talk with other kids your age whose parents are divorced, or with adults who understand."
• By being open to hearing reactions to the divorce. Questions will be answered by parents at depth when they are asked.	"We both still care about you very much. Mom and Dad's feelings for each other have changed, but not our feelings about you."
• By staying parental and protective, minimizing competition with child when both parent and child are dating.	"We both are dating, but I am still your mother."
• By minimizing adult emotional and physical dependency upon the child.	"No, don't stay home this evening because I am sad. I am okay and I want you to have a good time."
• By providing as stable a context as possible so that age-appropriate	"I'll be right here in case you need to call me for a ride."

separation-individuation may proceed.

• By recognizing that parent's acting out his or her own painful feelings is providing an example for child to act out feelings with substances, sexually, or through anti-social behavior.	"I did foul up last night and I feel bad about it. I want to be in control, and a good role-model for you."
• By recognizing the emotional vulnerability of the child who is in transition, realizing that divorce will add a risk factor to an already burdened child.	"I know it's tough to be handling junior high and the divorce all at once. There are special people to talk with who help with all of these changes."
• By recognizing the number of transitions involved in the divorce and moving to junior high school; helping the child to minimize other changes of home, neighborhood, peer groups where possible.	"Maybe we should put off the change in the weekend schedule until you feel more settled in our new house."
• By recognizing the impact of both parents suddenly needing to work and by providing consistent after school structure for the child.	"Mrs. Smythe is going to be at the house every day after school, making dinner. She'll be available to you if you need her."

Principles for Talking with Young Adults about Divorce	Examples of Principle
Parent helps child:	Parent says to child:
• By expressing confidence in child's various skills.	"You've learned some things by having your Mom and me in different places: like respect for different values, how to negotiate andpromise."

• By expressing the belief that child is separate from them and need not follow the same divorce course.	"My hope for you is that, at the right time, you will find someone very special to marry and with whom to have a family."
• By expressing faith in child's ability to persevere in work and academically in spite of the crisis of divorce.	"I know it is very hard to hang in there with your studies and activities, but I believe you can do it."
• By being aware that child may believe that marriage is a sham, that many years of marriage and raising children was meaningless, that the young adult's ability to trust himself or herself in relationships may be impaired.	"I still believe in marriage. Just because Dad's and my marriage didn't last forever doesn't mean that you won't be able to have a lasting relationship."
• By being able to accept no for an answer when: - asking young adult for information about the other parent - asking the child to function with the parent in a surrogate spouse's position, - asking young adult to meet parent's needs which would curtail the young person's own developmental progress.	"I respect your right to say no. You shouldn't have to be put in the middle between your mother and me."

This table was created collaboratively by Judith Ashway, LICSW clinical social work private practitioner in Belmont, Massachusetts; Rita Van Tassel, LICSW clinical social work private practitioner in Brookline, Massachusetts; and Janet Miller Wiseman LICSW clinical social work private practitioner in Lexington, Massachusetts.

9

Selection of Clients

A colleague asked me whether I put all couple clients coming to me into mediation therapy, adding "I'll bet you do!" I was grateful for the question. I thought carefully about my initial phone call with all clients, during which I spell out the differences in the approaches for which they might be candidates. In many of my colleagues' minds, the difference between couples therapy and marriage counseling is that the former is thought to be a place to work on the entity between them, their relationship, with the goal of improving it. Couples therapy is frequently thought to be of indefinite duration, while marriage counseling may also be of indefinite duration but is thought to frequently include a decision-making component about whether the relationship can last, before beginning work on communication, sexual, and/or parenting issues.

As I have repeated many times in this book, in contrast to

couples therapy and similar in one way to many clinicians' notions of marriage counseling, mediation therapy is a very highly structured, time-limited intervention, the sole goal of which is to make a decision, often about the future direction of a relationship. Asking people to identify what their goals are, and where they believe they fit into a spectrum of interventions, gives all couple clients the power to be included in the decisionmaking process of which intervention suits them best. Rather than lumping all couple clients into mediation therapy, I believe I am more acutely aware of empowering prospective clients to think with me about what their needs are and how those needs will be served by a particular therapeutic intervention.

The Ideal Candidates

When asked about the ideal candidates for mediation therapy, I say that the candidates who have the easiest time in using mediation therapy are the people with healthy personality structures who have heard about the intervention from a therapist, or a lawyer, or a friend, and have already determined for themselves that

this approach is for them. Qualities of such a healthy personality are:

intelligence

an ability to delay making decisions and the achievement
of gratification

a strong ability to distinguish outside reality from one's
own internal reality

an ability to tolerate ambiguity

an ability to see oneself clearly, with a sense of humor an ability to

make good judgments
verbal expressiveness

Such a person, at the extreme, may not need mediation therapy. However, this is a

clinical intervention that is primarily a decision-making intervention; it is appropriate

for even very healthy personalities and less appropriate for very unhealthy personalities.

Interestingly, some of the attributes of the healthy personality might also be liabilities. Intelligence, when it turns into intellectualization, can be a barrier to knowing one's self in all of one's aspects. Of Carl Jung's four psychological styles (intuition, thinking, feeling, sensation), it might appear that the person with the intuitive mode might optimally use mediation therapy. In my observation, many intuitive people may readily come to a decision about a future direction, but considerable numbers have difficulty sustaining certainty in their decisions. Being able to ground intuition in the rational understanding of a decision and in sensory information and instructional information is an ideal.

One of many advantages of having a clinician, and not a nontherapist mediator be the facilitator of mediation therapy is that screening for the process is highly important. When asked who the worst candidates are for the process, I respond by saying that those people who, for whatever reason, have little capacity to observe themselves are impossible candidates for mediation therapy. Those who are very distrusting, thought-disordered, paranoid, or with any type of psychosis or untreated major affective disorder are most generally *not* candidates for mediation therapy. Also, when a client is unable to share the mediation therapist with a spouse or where one person is involved in a hidden affair or a flagrantly insensitive open affair, mediation therapy is not indicated. When one person has a hidden agenda, knowing he or she will separate or divorce, but who wants to have the mediation therapy look like an honest attempt at saving the relationship, the mediation therapy will not work as it is constructed to work. In my experience, when there is hidden, not open, homosexuality, the process will be almost always aborted. In addition, those Catch-22 situations where a husband says to his wife, "I will leave my lover of seven years, if you'll promise to take me back" and she says "There is no way I'll take you back, until you've quit seeing her for six months," are impossible to work with positively in mediation therapy at this stage because of the draw between the partners.

Attempting to ascertain which individuals in classic diagnostic categories can use mediation therapy is difficult. Qualities such as adequate ability to observe oneself may be present in a person seen as having a high-functioning borderline personality disorder or in someone with a unipolar depression, which is being treated psychopharmacologically. Severe disorders of any type, thought disorders, affective disorders, personality disorders, active addictive disorders most likely would be contraindications to an effective usage of mediation therapy. Yet there are always exceptions. A woman called, referred by her and her husband's psychotherapist, saying that they both had "quite serious character disorders," but that their couples therapist thought they could do mediation therapy. The intensity of anger within the mediation therapy and between sessions was extraordinary, but they made a caring and mature decision to separate in the process.

Active alcoholism that is being completely denied makes mediation therapy, in my

experience, impossible to do from sessions one to twelve. People have gone into

detoxification and alcohol treatment programs almost immediately after coming for

mediation therapy and returned later for decision making, along with attending Co-

dependents, Alcoholics Anonymous, Narcotics Anonymous, or Gamblers Anonymous,

and Al-Anon meetings. When alcohol or another substance is impairing a person's

judgment and personality to any degree, mediation therapy is not, in my experience,

an appropriate intervention. My students of mediation therapy, who have been

workers and specialists in substance abuse treatment, however, claim that mediation

therapy may be well adapted for families of recovering alcoholics and substance

users. In fact, Robyn Ferrero has written about using mediation therapy for the

codependent spouse and the recovering alcoholic.[1] Because the values advocated in

mediation therapy are also fundamental to

—

352

the treatment of co-dependency, Ferrero determines that mediation therapy may

be adapted for co-dependents. As well as espousing honesty, both treatments

discourage the use of blaming, manipulation and dualistic thinking.

Ferrero, who refers to the work of Anne Wilson Schaef, attributes the

efficacy of mediation therapy with co-dependents to the idea that the individuals,

as well as the mediation therapist, are in charge of the process.[2] She states, "Since

a major characteristic of the disease of alcoholism is controlling, a counselor modeling

controlling behavior reinforces the disease of co-dependency." Mediation therapy, in

contrast, gives control to the clients by encouraging them to come to their own

decisions, guided but not overly influenced by a neutral third party.

According to Ferrero, mediation therapy may be adapted for use with co-dependents,

provided the mediation therapist understands the characteristics of co-dependency

and is free of

bias [see Appendix C for an alcohol use bias sorter]. In addition, Ferrero states, the

mediation therapist must understand the issues facing co-dependents, including the

need to establish strong self-identity apart from the partner^ and the necessity of

defining boundaries between the self and others. In Ferrero's view, the mediation

therapist must be particularly aware not only of the conflicts between the co-

dependent and the recovering alcoholic, but of those between the co-dependent and

his or her own disease. For mediation therapy to be beneficial, Ferrero also believes

that mediation therapy is most useful for individuals who recognize their

codependency.

The goals of the co-dependent may be the goals anyone else would have in the

intervention, or they may be something like, "My goal is to learn to carry on positively

with my own life, regardless of the drinking or non-drinking behavior of my

spouse." Combining my own view that active alcoholism is not the best state in which

to conduct mediation therapy, with Ferrero's thesis that mediation therapy is a

natural approach for

the partners of alcoholics or substance abusers, results in the conclusion that substance abusers in recovery, along with their codependent spouses, may well show themselves to be very effective users of mediation therapy.[3]

—

Students of mediation therapy have advised me to build into my initial screening telephone call normalized questions about alcohol use in the extended family, saying, "To what extent is alcohol or drug use a problem in your family?" Time and experience will show how this question may shape the mediation therapy process or may influence clients' decisions to use a more direct intervention for the alcohol or drug problem itself.

A Growing Role for Mediation Therapy

Occasionally people inquire about what the positives are in mediation therapy. I sometimes share with them (carefully disguised) case examples. I tell them that in my observation, when people are provided with a serious, safe, structured forum in which they are offered tools with which to make critically important decisions, that they often very rapidly take more responsibility for themselves than they heretofore imagined undertaking. Their potential for tolerating indecision and taking a comprehensive look at their lives gives them, I believe, a sense of mastery and integrity. Although the sole goal of the process is making a decision, positive behavioral changes and attitudinal shifts in individuals are as notable as I have seen in any other form of psychotherapy. Individuals' ego-functioning often improves; they seem to verbalize more, and act out their feelings less—for example, deciding about the future of their marriage rather than starting an affair that would likely lead to the demise of the marriage. Emotionally intense feelings are discharged within a safe structure, in the mediation therapy. Children's needs during the mediation therapy are focused upon and not overlooked, giving parents a sense of mastery and a feeling of responsibility that they are continuing to care for the precious products of their union.

Caring for these children whose parents are in crisis, separating, and divorcing, as well as those who have special educational needs, is sometimes accomplished within school meetings in educational plan evaluations. Judith Field, a student of mediation therapy who chairs a special needs evaluation team in Greater Boston, spoke of adapting mediation therapy in a school setting for children with special needs.[4] Field found that prior to a special needs evaluation team meeting, parents, educators, and students harbored high levels of anxiety. By asking the parents to think about their goals for the team meeting in advance, they don't come into the meeting unsure of what they want to accomplish. The phone call prior to the meeting, in which the educator talks with both parents, eases their nervousness, and helps them collect important information and articulate their concerns. The sixteen- to eighteen-year-old student whose educational plan is being discussed, is, of course, also met with to express his or her goals for an educational plan.

He or she is included in the process that determines his or her life very directly. The classroom teacher and guidance counselor are also asked their goals for the team meeting, as is the director of the special needs program, who needs to develop goals that are within the program's budget.

When the team meeting begins, the special needs advocate articulates or has the individuals themselves articulate their goals for the meeting. He or she assumes responsibility for keeping the discussion focused on the goals so that it doesn't end in an explosive outcome, with no resolution. Prior to the team meeting the staff meets to brainstorm alternatives for each student. The perspectives of the student and the parents are taken into consideration. When the technical assessment reports are given in the meeting, they are rephrased and reframed so that parents and students understand the implications. During the meeting, paraphrasing, active listening, and brainstorming are used to facilitate the planning process. Judith Field has adapted some of the mediation therapy principles creatively for use with children in an educational planning setting. In a similar way, the mediation

therapy principles may be adapted for use in a variety of settings.

Mediation therapy is being used by nursing home staffs, in inpatient psychiatric units,

in the guidance departments of high schools, in drug education programs, in prisons,

and in other settings. One student of mediation therapy who works with couples in a

prison, commented that my conflict skills were not originally designed for use with

prisoners. However, through the mediation therapy course, he designed an eight-

session process that would help couples determine mutual goals while one

partner was in prison. He discovered a recurring pattern in these couples. Frequently,

the man felt disempowered and helpless while in prison, while the wife felt

resentment and anger about parenting alone. He found that couples very

frequently developed similar goals for themselves: the wives wanted to be able to ask

for and trust their husbands' input about parenting the children and running the

house; and the husbands wanted

their wives to trust them enough to ask for help and advice about the children and running the household.

When colleagues ask just how mediation therapy differs from other time-limited, solution-focused, or cognitive approaches, I answer that it may be more similar than different. Its uniqueness may be in its organization and blend of attitudes and techniques that are widely used in other interventions. It is different from some approaches, and the same as still other interventions—in its use of instruction, that is, of psychoeducational material. Time is taken to teach people to be assertive, to communicate well, to negotiate on a sophisticated level, to disagree effectively and to make important decisions. Couples in mediation therapy are strongly aware that their facilitator is trained to be neutral between them. This neutrality is made more explicit in mediation therapy than I believe it to be in other interventions. In mediation therapy, the values of the mediation therapist are made explicit. These values are not passed off as conventional wisdom or research findings, but as the mediation therapist's own values. In mediation therapy the attitudinal stance of the facilitator is that of expert, not authority. That is, the mediation therapist has an area of expertise to share with the couple or family, but is distinctly not about to pass judgment on the couple or advise them directly what to do.

Applications of the mediation therapy process are many. One clinician is teaching it to other clinicians on an inpatient psychiatric unit. She especially wants to reduce the over identification of staff with the patient in the hospital. She is attempting to increase staff members' neutrality so that they may help their patients understand the feelings and needs of their family members, who are frequently overextending themselves due to the hospitalization process. It is all too easy to make the patient in the hospital the victim of family members' insensitivity.

Another clinician, working in a nursing home, is using mediation therapy to help staff and family become more united in the interests of the elderly person. She believes that family is often "grieving the loss of function, and anticipating the death of their family member."[5] She believes the family often feels guilty about the institutionalization, as well as anxiety about dwindling financial resources. Over those things, they have no control. They can, however, attempt to control and supervise the staff of the nursing home. Of course, the staff interprets the supervision by patients' family members as lack of confidence in their competence, as criticism, and as unnecessary control. The supervision often stemmed from families' feelings of helplessness. Mediation therapy or techniques from it are used by this clinician, who, as a neutral, helps staff and family members understand each other's goals and who attempts to "help them forge a bond for the sake of the patient."[6]

Another clinician is using mediation therapy in a high school, where she is attempting to gain neutral status, even though the initial person she invariably sees is a young person, who is often severely at odds with his or her parents.

For years, a fellow clinician has been using the mediation therapy approach with families of patients on an organ transplant and dialysis unit in a hospital. Sorting through her own biases about critical health issues, she has found it imperative to be neutral in helping family members make decisions about their loved ones.

As previously stated, the approach lends itself particularly well to couples attempting to make decisions about marriage or living together. Because they don't have years of experience, entrenched negative patterns of interaction, and extensive knowledge about their partnership, adherence to the mediation therapy format in a more structured fashion is often appropriate. Searching through mediation therapy cases to find interesting ones to use for illustration, I invariably picked those in which couples were making a decision to live together or to marry, because they showed the format in such a "pure form."

The approach has also been very effective with parents and

college-attending children, and those who are about to leave college, in clarifying the extent of their financial, filial, and emotional responsibilities to one another.

Business partners have used the approach to clarify the parameters of their partnership and whether they want to continue the partnership.

Wherever two people, two groups, or two organizations desire to determine a joint direction, there may be applicability for mediation therapy.

Taking a look at which psychotherapists might or might not be eligible to do mediation therapy is to witness a self-selection process. Just how much does a therapist's own relationship or marriage history impact on his or her ability to be a neutral mediation therapist? Can mediation therapists who have not been divorced facilitate a process that results in divorce? Do divorced mediation therapists always advocate divorce for their clients?

Ostensibly, all mediation therapists will have examined their biases so that they are aware of them and can be neutral about others' decisions regardless of their own marital status. They may be biased, but they are also trained to be neutral.

There have been several students of mediation therapy who have determined that, due to their religious or cultural beliefs in the permanence of marriage, they could not act as mediation therapists for couples trying to make a separation, divorce, or remain-together decision. Those same therapists saw themselves as being useful mediation therapists where there were other types of decisions to be made. As previously stated, being aware of one's biases is critical to becoming an effective neutral. If, to mention a previous case, a mediation therapist felt her marriage ended partially as a result of an eighteen-year difference in ages, taking on a couple with a large age difference might well be thoughtfully considered before proceeding with mediation therapy.

People whose track records with marriage have been very discouraging, but who have found success in living together in an intimate relationship, may find helping a young couple make a commitment to marriage somewhat difficult. It is inevitable that one's own experiences impact one's belief system about relationships. It is fundamental to understand one's biases about relationships, and where and whether they impact on one's abilities to work with certain couples or families in mediation therapy or, even whether they may preclude being a neutral mediation therapist.

Mediation Therapy and Gender

Jurg Willi's *Couples in Collusion* includes some very interesting research relating to gender roles and the responses of women and men when they are alone and together.

Using the Individual and the Common Rorschach tests, Willi measured men's and women's responses when they are alone and when they are in one another's presence. He found that in single testing sessions, women demonstrated constructive approaches to a working relationship, while in couples testing sessions they tended to behave more regressively and passively. They held themselves back, waited for the approval of men, inhibited their ego responses, failed to see the overall picture.

Men spoke openly about their weaknesses in single testing sessions, while in couples sessions they tended to suppress responses to images that suggested emotion, sexual impulses, inner conflicts, sensitivity, anxiety, depressing moods. They became more active, more decisive, and more persistent when they reacted to women in a couples situation than when they were alone.

In many of my own sessions, women and men exhibit these differences. A woman who was an expressive interpreter for the deaf animatedly described how things could be different in her marriage. When she and I met with her husband, she exhibited no hand motion in the session, and had inhibited speech and a depressed affect. Willi found that in a couples situation women restricted their own overviews of situations, abdicated to their husbands, became less productive, withheld themselves more emotionally and relinquished a sense of reality. Willi's experience with the Common Rorschach and in couples therapy showed "that women have a tendency to live below their potential and to relinquish their self-realization in a couple relationship."[7]

—

On the man's part, Willi's findings showed that men tend to feel that if they openly admit to feelings of insecurity and weakness that they will transfer power to their wives. It is Willi's assertion that when a man suppresses his own anxiety, weakness, or guilt, he is also unable to perceive his partner's feelings. Indeed, Willi found that men and women presented different personalities depending upon whether they were with their spouses or alone.[8]

—

Some of the goals of couples therapy as seen by Willi are "to loosen up, de-emphasize very rigid interactional personalities, to react less strongly to the personality of the other partner, develop 'relative individuation,' experiencing themselves as separate from and relative to one another."[9] Many of the rational structures of mediation therapy, which focus on the uniqueness of individuals, tend to support one of the central goals of Willi's couple therapy: "that the man and woman overcome this self-alienation, 'retrieve their selves' and develop two separate yet mutually relating personalities—but not personalities which are determined through mutual influence"[10].

Willi's description of the relative differences in gender behavior when men and women are together and his goals for couples therapy are instructive for mediation therapists. Therapists need to be aware that the behavior of their couple clients, while together, may differ markedly from their behavior when they are alone. The fact that one's own gender may play a role in the mediation therapy needs to be acknowledged by the mediation therapist and discussed with the couple when appropriate. The mediation therapist's emphasis on synthesizing rationality and emotionality is an attempt to help each partner participate in what may be the other's dominant approach to understanding.

One group of mediation therapy students concurred that women feel more helped by women therapists, while men feel more helped by men therapists. But what about those women who identify with men, and who believe men to be more effective? Or those women who saw their mothers as being incompetent, so similarly view a female therapist? Do some men see all women as potentially undermining or protecting or seducing them? What implications might these gender assumptions have for mediation therapy, or any therapy, for that matter? Does it happen that when a couple uses a female mediation therapist, that the man, in the presence of his own female partner and the female mediation therapist, becomes doubly ego-expansive, doubly inhibiting his vulnerable responses? Does the situation provoke the female partner to be less ego-expansive (less masterful in my terms), and to depend on her partner more for describing their situation, but less so than if the mediation therapist were a man? At minimum, we need to be aware that our genders, our styles, may provoke somewhat uncharacteristic responses that would not be there, in the same degree, if we weren't there.

The positive aspects of marriage as seen by Willi are "that the ego must expand at marriage to consider the spouse as well as the self and also the marriage as an entity."[11] Both partners ideally come to see "that their partner's *individuality* broadens their own experience and that separateness too is a part of love."[12] Willi quotes Theodore Lidz: "A successful marriage will generally lead to and require a profound reorganization of the personality structure of each partner that will influence the further personality development of each."[13] Willi and Lidz highlight here an opportunity for couples in crisis; either to recognize the potential they have to grow as individuals and as an entity or to recognize an inevitability to their parting. Crisis and opportunity are interchangeable in mediation therapy.

Outcomes of Mediation Therapy

What are the sorts of outcomes achieved by mediation therapy? They reflect the unique needs, values, and desires of every couple or family using mediation therapy. Some people stay in relationships that appear supportive. Others remain in relationships that don't appear to support the individuals adequately, but who report back, years later, on the richness of their relationships and express gratitude that they persevered. Many people choose to separate or divorce through the process; some make mutual decisions, some mutually understood decisions, and some nonmutual decisions. Some people stage their decisions over time: "We will live together for a year, then determine whether to become engaged or to part," or, "We will separate for a year, checking in exactly in one year to see whether we should work on a divorce, attempt a reconciliation, or continue the separation."

Who makes the decision for the couple in mediation therapy? When my son, Todd, now nineteen, was nine years old, I took him and his Israeli friend Hedva to buy a Christmas tree. Enroute I began to cry. Both children were solicitous, wondering what the matter could be. Todd offered it was something about my work. I admitted I was sad that a truly wonderful couple I had been working with had just terminated their work with me. Then I added, "I feel sad that I wasn't able to save their marriage." My son, in the best psychiatric consult I ever had said, "Mom, you're only their little helper, they make the big decision."

Our clients, not us, make the decision about the future direction of their lives. We carefully guide, even control the process, but our clients make the ultimate decision, taking both the responsibility and the credit for their decisions. Initially, mediation therapists may experience a wide variety of feelings at the point when their clients decide the future direction of their relationship: feeling like a destroyer of marriages, a failure as a therapist, or feeling overly responsible for any decision are only a few of the feelings, or countertransference reactions, that may come as a result of a couple's or a family's making a decision.

If the mediation therapist remembers that she or he is only their "little helper" while they truly make the big decision, then she or he has provided them with a sophisticated forum in which to make their decisions. She or he has not made the decisions for them, and can take neither the responsibility, nor the blame, nor the credit for the decisions that have been made. The mediation therapist will have had the honor of being present with couples and families at momentous crossroads in their lives, while mediation therapy clients will have had the benefit of a sane, safe, structured process that guides them out of conflict and into important next stages of their lives.

Notes

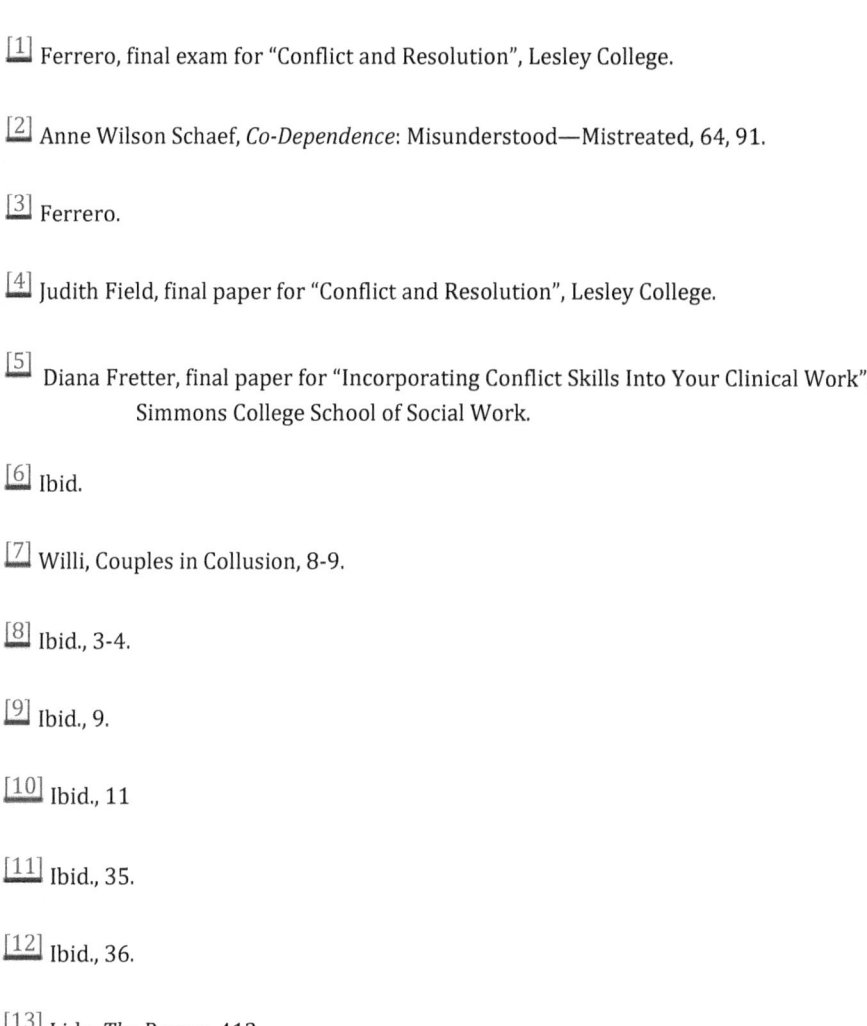

[1] Ferrero, final exam for "Conflict and Resolution", Lesley College.

[2] Anne Wilson Schaef, *Co-Dependence*: Misunderstood—Mistreated, 64, 91.

[3] Ferrero.

[4] Judith Field, final paper for "Conflict and Resolution", Lesley College.

[5] Diana Fretter, final paper for "Incorporating Conflict Skills Into Your Clinical Work", Simmons College School of Social Work.

[6] Ibid.

[7] Willi, Couples in Collusion, 8-9.

[8] Ibid., 3-4.

[9] Ibid., 9.

[10] Ibid., 11

[11] Ibid., 35.

[12] Ibid., 36.

[13] Lidz, *The Person*, 412.

Distribution of Structures in Mediation

Therapy

Students of mediation therapy frequently ask where rational, emotional, sensory, and instructional structures are placed within the time-limited mediation therapy structure. Sensitive and creative mediation therapists will not rigidly adhere to a predesigned format. Clients have their own agendas, and flexibility on the part of the mediation therapist is necessary in order to meet their needs. I include, nonetheless, this chart, which outlines a basic structure that I follow in the twelvesession format. I encourage people to adapt or modify this format to meet the genuine needs of their clients.

Session One

· Explanation of the process

· Couples' individual goals for the intervention (rational

structure number one)

· Couples' theories about the breakdown or impasse in the relationship (rational structure number two)

· Couples' family of origin's perception of their crisis (rational structure number three)

· Impertinent questions (rational structure number four)

· Each individual's main internal issue (rational structure number six)

· Explanations and forms given for essential lists (rational structure number five)

Session Two

· Thoughts and feelings prompted by and evoked after session one, that is, the couple's agenda from session one

· Essential lists alternately read and discussed, hypotheses made, interpersonal work outlined

· Synopsis of their answers to rational structures one through six given by therapist and discussed with couple

Session Three

· Their agenda from session two

· Comparison of first several years (or months) of
  relationship, with last several years (or months), and stages in
between (rational structure number seven)

· The repetitive patterns in the couple's relationship; their
  "poulet-oeuf" questions (rational structure
  number ten)

· The positives in the relationship   (rational structure
  number eight)

· Sensory instruction to keep eyes, ears, intuition open to
  the realities of their relationship, themselves, the other

· Instruction in and distribution of geneogram forms
  (rational structure number twelve)

Session Four

· Their agenda from session three

· Their *geneograms* talked about   (rational structure
        number twelve)

· Mini-training in assertiveness · Mini-

training in communication
· What strong feelings do they have at the present time
        about anyone or anything?

· Homework assignments given in assertiveness and
        communication training

Session Five

· Their agenda from session four, including any examples
        of good, assertive communication

· Instruction in negotiation and in disagreement

· The aches, gripes, conflicts, anxieties between them
        (rational structure number eleven)

· Are those aches a threat to the relationship?

Session Six

· Their agenda from session five ·

Instruction in decision making

· Highlighting by mediation therapist that this is the

midpoint of their process; they are gathering, gestating, considering much information

· Summary by clients of what they have learned

· Summary by mediation therapist of what they have

discovered

· Assessment by therapist of whether couple is beginning

to implement what they have learned, whether their affects are depressed, energetic, labile

Session Seven

· Their agenda from session six

· Taking and arguing each other's initial position about the

relationship

· How are their children doing? What do they need?

Sharing experience and research about children's

needs during parental crisis (rational structure number nineteen)

· Ascertaining how well they are communicating, negotiating

· Teaching effective disagreement

· Listing of their objectives for mediation therapy, their alternative future directions and considerations for making a decision. Correlating options with objectives and considerations.

Session Eight

· Their agenda from session seven · Beginning

instruction in forgiveness
· What have the negatives been in the relationship, for the self or for the other? (rational structure number nine)

· Can they begin to forgive one another for the negatives and the hurts in the relationship?

· Their assessment of their own ability to change; how

        able are they to compromise versus how intractable are

their difficulties, patterns, conflicts?

Session Nine

    · Their agenda from session eight

    · Clarification of all past misunderstandings and asking of

        forgiveness (rational structure number fourteen)

    · Mediation therapist's talk about the power of decision

        making and about the data they are gathering to grow those

decisions. The benefits to all concerned of mutually made or

understood decisions, not unilateral decisions (rational

        structure number thirteen)

Session Ten

    · Their agenda from session nine

    · Emphasis made that two more sessions remain · Mediation therapist asks

that individuals be aware of all

around them, using all their senses, and become aware that an integration of the rational, emotional, sensory selves has been underway for some time

Session Eleven

· Their agenda from session ten

· Sharing from the heart with one another (rational structure number sixteen)

· How will they feel when decision is made about future direction of their relationship?

· Some people will share their decisions (rational structure number seventeen)

· What have they learned from one another that they will carry forward into the future? (rational structure number fifteen)

Session Twelve

· Their agenda from session eleven and all previous sessions permeates the session

383

· Individual decisions shared and negotiated to mutually

        understood or declared oppositional decisions (rational structure

number eighteen)

· Discussion of implementation of decisions, future

        therapy, legal/mediation planning, planning for children's,

elders' needs (rational structures

        number nineteen and twenty)

The Twenty Rational Structures

1. What are each individual's separate goals for the intervention?

2. What are each individual's theories about the breakdown or impasse in the relationship?

3. How does each individual think their family of origin (FOO) or other significant parenting figures would view their relationship crisis if they knew everything that the individual knows about it?

4. The Impertinent questions:[1]   ▬

   · What attracted you to your partner (your mate, your spouse) in the first place?

   · What do you presently like the most about your partner?

   · What did your partner bring to your unit that you lacked at the time you got together? Which of these characteristics still contrast with your own characteristics?

· What would you miss most about your partner if the
two of you should ever decide to part?

· What presently bothers you most about your partner?

· What do you presently need, want, or count on from
your mate that you could or would like to do for yourself?

· Do you see yourselves as being similar, as true
opposites to one another, or just on opposite ends of the same
continuum (that is, both having trouble with control, but one partner
being overly neat and the other partner overly messy)?

· Are the difficulties between you recent and acute or
are they longstanding? Are they a threat to the relationship?

· What fears, if any, do you have about being alone or
not in the relationship should you part?

· Trace your major fights. What were the overt and

underlying causes?

· What skills do you still desire to learn from your
partner?

· What are the factors that tie you together? 5. The
essential lists:

· What do you know you want and need in any good
long-term relationship?

· What do you know you cannot tolerate in any good
long-term relationship?

· What do you bring as problems/difficulties to any good
long-term relationship?

· What do you bring as strengths to any good long-term
relationship?

6. What main internal issue is each person dealing with
right now?

7. How do the first several years, or months, of the relationship
compare with the last several years, or months? Were there identifiable
stages in

between?

8. What positives have there been in the relationship?

    Which remain today?

9. What negatives have there been in the relationship?

    Which remain today?

10. What are the repetitive patterns in the relationship?

    The poulet-oeuf (chicken-or-the-egg) questions?

11. What are the collective issues in the relationship?

    Which aches, gripes, conflicts, and anxieties would need to be resolved for the couple to have a rewarding relationship?

12. The geneogram depicting how the individuals'

    extended families have handled conflict.

13. Instruction in the importance of mutually understood,

    if not mutually agreed-upon, decisions.

14. Clarification of past misunderstandings and asking of

    forgiveness.

15. What will individuals carry forward into the future,

whether living together or not?

16. An emotional sharing from the heart and a rational listing of alternative future directions.

17. Individual decisions reported; negotiation to mutual or mutually understood decisions.

18. A negotiated settlement between the two individual decisions.

19. Information about children's needs during crisis.

20. Planning the next steps after the negotiated settlement.

[1] The impertinent questions (item 4) were devised primarily by Priscilla Bonney Smith.

Marriage and Divorce

1. Do you believe in marriage? What is it? What is commitment? Axe they the same?

2. Do you believe in marital separation? Under certain circumstances? And not under other circumstances?

3. Do you believe in divorce? Under certain circumstances and not under others?

4. What religious, cultural, general background views, past and present, do you hold about divorce or marriage?

5. When couples have children, does that at all influence your opinion about whether couples should stay together?

6. Do children fare better in intact families with unhappily married couples, than in divorced families with

happily divorced parents?

7. How do you feel about gay and lesbian relationships? Are you at all uncomfortable in the presence of these couples?

8. How do you feel about interracial or intercultural relationships (for example a black man and a white woman; a Russian man and an American woman)? Are you uncomfortable in the presence of these couples?

9. How do you feel about relationships in which there is a large difference in age?

10. How do you feel about relationships in which one person has a physical handicap, a mental disability, or AIDS?

11. What is your own current image of a healthy relationship?

12. Do you believe in living together on a long-term or shortterm basis without marriage?

1. Do you like or enjoy conflict? 2. Do you

hate or avoid conflict?

3. Is it easier to help others manage their conflicts than for
you to deal directly with your own conflicts?

4. How did your family of origin handle conflict?

5. How much more effectively do you want to handle
conflict between yourself and others, personally and
professionally?

Gender

1. Are either men or women better able to make
decisions?

2. Are women (or men) more able to express themselves
in therapy?

3. Are men more rational than women? 4. Are women

more emotional than men?
5. Do you believe you can empathize better with a

member of the same sex?

6. Do you believe you can stay neutral, not siding with or
   against someone of the same (or opposite) sex?

7. Can you put aside your own beliefs about how the
   gender roles in a relationship should work?

Hospitals/Hospices

Most of these questions were created by Sue Oberbeck-Friedlich,
LICSW, medical social worker at the Deaconness Hospital in
Boston, and social worker in private practice in Boston.

1. Do you believe in organ donation?

2. Should sick people go directly from the hospital to adult
   children's homes to live, especially if there will be probable
   dislocation and disruption of family members?

3. Do you believe in nursing homes for people who could
   be cared for by others at home?

4. Should everyone hear his or her diagnosis? When
   should diagnoses be withheld?

5. Does a spouse have the responsibility to care for the ill

person at his or her own vocational, or physical or mental health

expense?

6. Should a couple stay married if all financial resources

will be drained from one to care for the other, who is a sick person

institutionalized for many years and for the most part is incommunicative ?

7. Should resuscitation always be attempted?

8. Are there cases in which you believe in withdrawal of

life- supports?

9. Do you tell someone they are off (or on) the waiting list

for the donation of an organ?

Alcohol

This bias sorter was designed by Lynne Yansen, LICSW, a social worker in private practice in Lexington, Massachusetts and at Harvard Health Plan in Peabody, Massachusetts; and by the Norcap Inpatient Detoxification Unit staff at Southwood Community Hospital, Norfolk, Massachusetts and Jan Schwartz, MSW, Ed.D., psychotherapist in private practice in Brookline, Massachusetts.

1. What is your definition of an alcoholic? Is alcohol abuse

alcoholism? How do you distinguish alcohol abuse from

alcoholism? From moderate social drinking?

2. What is your definition of social drinking?

3. Do you believe that alcoholism is inherited? Does it run
in families?

4. Do you adhere to the disease concept of alcoholism? If
not, how do you conceptualize alcoholism?

5. Can recovering alcoholics become social drinkers? 6. Does a person need

to drink daily to be an alcoholic? 7. What is your view of an alcoholic?

Describe the person.

8. Do you know of alcoholism in your own extended
family?

9. Is it OK for people to drink to relax or reduce stress? 10. When should

people drink?

11. How much do you drink?

12. Is there a difference in what one drinks as to his or her

potential for alcoholism? What is the difference between drinking beer, wine, or whiskey?

13. If a person works or functions every day, would you consider him or her not to be alcoholic?

14. Can professionals such as doctors, judges, lawyers, corporate executives, be alcoholic?

15. Should people who are actively drinking engage in couples therapy? Mediation therapy?

16. Are newly recovering alcoholics and their families prepared for a therapeutic intervention? How long after sobriety is achieved will couples be prepared to begin a therapeutic intervention?

17. What does alcoholism say about the morality of the alcoholic?

Stages of a Couple Relationship

Couple relationships may evolve in many ways. I describe here one possibility for the evolution of a couple relationship.

Blind Attraction. *Basic theme*: Falling in love, feeling terrific, idealizing the other as part of the self, ignoring or denying any weaknesses, negative traits, faults. Judgment may be impaired and self-esteem enhanced by feeling understood, and making a good "catch." A feeling of oneness, merger, occurs when dependency needs are being fulfilled, without the threat of loss of self.

Temporarily Removing the Blindfold. *Basic theme*: Becoming aware of behaviors, character traits that challenge original perceptions of the other. A disregarding or minimizing of these latter perceptions may occur in order to keep the original infatuation intact.

Casting off the Blindfold. *Basic theme*: Disappointment, anger, feelings of letdown and loss occur when the original vision of the relationship doesn't match the reality and it can no longer be ignored: the partner and the relationship simply are not as flawless and made in heaven as originally viewed. There may be the beginnings of desires to devalue the other when the vision of the good, even ideal partnership is blown away, and when needs— legitimate or extraordinary—are not being fulfilled as expected through the relationship.

Lashing Out. *Basic theme*: The partner is seen as the cause of one's disappointment and feelings of being let-down, and is thought of as weak or human, or even as malicious, deplorable: the enemy. Interactions are tense, conflictual, even hostile. Partners struggle against each other and for power and control of one another, the relationship, their children, their work, and so forth.

Retreating. *Basic theme*: Fear of further loss and disruption causes partners to retreat from their hostilities into jobs, children, friends, perhaps even lovers, which may defuse the intensity between them. However, there remains a feeling of disappointment and anger overridden by the need for security and continuity.

The Retreat Solidified. *Basic theme*: The roles that developed to avert separation and loss now become a way of life. The individuals take on separate identities and live quite separate lives, still not acknowledging their internal and interpersonal loss. They find contentment in various degrees in their individual activities and begin to realize that their original vision of a partnership and expectation of the other will not be fulfilled.

Mourning the Vision. *Basic theme*: Individuals arrive at a recognition that their visions and expectations will not be met with the partner, nor with anyone. An understanding arises that needs must be fulfilled within the self. Initially, individuals experience sadness and loss. That loss gradually becomes transformed into a feeling of power that comes with the ability to be autonomous and with the giving up of the illusion of the need for dependence. People become more aware of the relationship as consisting of two separate individuals, and begin to enjoy the other as he or she is and are more able to appreciate differentness, rather than feeling threatened by it.

Re-Vision. *Basic theme*: Individuals are finally prepared to own one hundred percent responsibility for themselves, not depending on the other to intuit or fulfill their needs. They have learned to ask directly for help when they need it. Knowing they could choose to live alone or together, they choose to see and enjoy the strengths of the other. Individuals see and accept the partner, and place the partner's negative qualities in perspective. Paradoxically, partners alternate depending upon one another, with taking charge for the partnership. They make requests of the other and let go of the demand that these requests be honored. They are individuals who can be interdependent without being caught in overdependence.

These stages of a couple relationship were devised by Janet Miller Wiseman and Annette Kurtz, with reference to Simon and Glorianne Wittes' *Developmental Stages of a Couple Relationship*, which referred to *Becoming a Couple* by Roslyn Schwartz and Leonard J. Schwartz, a book published in 1980 by Prentice Hall.

Bandler, Richard, and John Grinder. *Frogs into Princes.* Moab, Utah: Real People Press, 1979.

Bazerman, Max. *Judgment in Managerial Decision Making.* New York: John Wiley & Sons, Inc., 1986.

Beck, Aaron. *Love Is Never Enough.* New York: Harper & Row, 1988.

Belenky, Mary Field, Blythe McVicker Clinchy, Nancy Rule Goldberger, and Jill Mattuck Tarule. *Women's Ways of Knowing.* New York: Basic Books, 1986.

Bernard, Yetta. *Conflict Resolution with a Couple.* Boston Family Institute: Perceptions Videotape Series, no date.

Bernard, Yetta. *Self-Care.* Millbrae, California; Celestial Arts, 1975. Casarjian,

Robin. *Forgiveness: A Bold Choice for a Peaceful Heart,* Bantum (in press).
____."Forgiveness Workshop." Watertown, MA,   1989. Sponsored by Interface, Watertown, MA.

Castenada, Carlos. *The Power of Silence.* New York: Simon & Schuster, 1987. "Census

Shows U.S. Family Households In Decline." *Boston Globe*, September 20, 1988.
Dawes, Robin, *Rational Choice in an Uncertain World.* San Diego: Harcourt, Brace, Jonanovich, San Diego, 1988.

Erikson, Joan M. *Wisdom and the Senses.* New York: W.W. Norton, 1988. Fanger,

Margot. "Strategic Brief Therapy." Massachusetts N.A.S.W.- sponsored workshop, North Andover MA, February 10, 1989. Ferrero, Robyn. Final paper for "Conflict and Resolution," Lesley College, summer 1989.

Field, Judith. Final paper for "Conflict and Resolution," Lesley College, summer 1989.

Fisher, Roger, and Scott Brown. *Getting Together: Building a Relationship That Gets to Yes.* Boston: Houghton Mifflin, 1988.

Fisher, Roger, and William Ury. *Getting to Yes: Negotiating Agreement Without Giving In.* Boston: Houghton Mifflin, 1981.

Gorman, Ira. "Decision Making Workshop." Portland, Connecticut, 1990 (unpublished workshop)

Greenwald, Harold. *Decision Therapy.* New York: Peter H. Wyden, 1973.

Grunebaum, Henry, Judith Christ, and Norman Nieburg. "Differential Diagnosis in the Treatment of Couples." Boston: unpublished paper, 1967.

Haley, Jay. *Problem-Solving Therapy*, 2d ed. San Francisco: Jossey-Bass,

1987. Langer, Ellen J. *Mindfulness.* Reading, MA: Addison-Wesley, 1989.
Lidz, Theodore. *The Person: His Development Throughout the Life Cycle.* New York: Basic Books, 1968.

Luepnitz, Deborah. "The Therapist and the Minotaur: Treating Men in Couples Therapy." Couples Therapy Conference, Harvard University, Continuing Education Program, October 21, 1989.

Mann, James. *Time-Limited Psychotherapy.* Cambridge: Harvard University Press, 1973.

Norton, Arthur J. and Moorman, Jeanne E., "Current Trends in Marriage and Divorce among American Women." *Journal of Marriage and the Family*, 49,1987: 3

14.

Poincare, Henri. "Intuition and Logic Mathematics." *Mathematics Teacher.* 62 (3), 1969: 205-212.

Roth, Sallyann, "Designing Tasks For Couples That Help Couples Continue Their Therapy At Home" Couples Therapy Conference, Harvard University, Continuing Education Program, October 21, 1989.

Rubin, Theodore Isaac. *Overcoming Indecisiveness: The Stages of Effective Decision Making.* New York: Harper & Row, 1985.

Sanford, John A. *Between People: Communicating One-to-One.* New York: Paulist Press, 1982.

Schaef, Anne Wilson. *Co-dependence: Misunderstood—Mistreated.* New York: Harper & Row, 1986.

Schwartz, Roslyn, and Leonard J. Schwartz. *Becoming a Couple.* Englewood Cliffs, N.J.: Prentice Hall, 1980.

Smith, Priscilla Bonney. "Mediation Therapy" exam. Lesley College, summer 1987.

Steinman, Susan, "The Experience of Children in the Joint-Custody Arrangement: A Report of a Study." *American Journal of Orthopsychiatry*, 51(3), July 1981: 403-414.

Wallerstein, Judith S., and Joan Kelly. *Surviving the Breakup: How Children and Parents Cope with Divorce.* New York: Basic Books, 1980.

Wallerstein, Judith S., and Sandra Blakeslee. *Second Chances: Men, Women and Children* a Decade After Divorce. New York: Ticknor & Fields, 1989.

Willi, Jurg. *Couples in Collusion.* New York: Jason Aronson,

1982.

Wittes, Simon and Glorianne. *Developmental Stages of a Couple Relationship.* Unpublished paper.

· collaborative mediation/mutual gains · interactive problem-

solving (basic human needs) · transformative mediation

· distributive bargaining

· decision making in mediation (mediation therapy) Ms. Miller Wiseman

consults to churches, temples,

hospitals, mental health centers, municipalities, schools and universities, prisons

and rehabilitation centers, dispute resolution centers. You may contact her at

Millerwise@aol.com or view the web page at www.mediationboston.com .

www.ingramcontent.com/pod-product-compliance
Lightning Source LLC
Chambersburg PA
CBHW051849170526
45168CB00001B/40